▬ THE EXPERTS PRAISE ▬
THE FAT-BURNING WORKOUT

"Whether you're an old pro or a beginner, you can use this book to burn the maximum fat and at the same time shape muscle."

—BEV FRANCIS
IFBB World Pro Bodybuilding Champion
author of *Bev Francis' Power Bodybuilding*

"The best workout I've seen yet for getting and staying in shape without a lot of wasted time and energy. I'll recommend this one to all of my patients—especially those who are endlessly dieting without permanent results. You burn fat, strengthen your heart and lungs—and at the same time reshape your body."

—JUDE BARBERA, M.D.
Assistant Clinical Professor of Surgery
Downstate Medical Center

"Your escape to freedom from fat—a super-program that works faster than any I've seen yet. You get the benefit of an aerobic workout while doing a bodybuilding routine."

—ANDY SIVERT
Mr. International and Mr. North America

"I recommend all of Joyce's books to my patients, because they provide the most effective workout with the least danger of injury. This one will be no exception."

—JACK BARNATHAN, D.C.
Director of Sports Health Chiropractic

"The super-giant set is a secret we bodybuilders have been using for years. Joyce has put it in simple language in *The Fat-Burning Workout,* so that anyone can understand and take advantage of it. So get with the program!"

—LINDA WOOD HOYTE
Masters USA Overall Champion

"It's a relief to read a book by a woman who practices what she preaches. Joyce is a role model for women half her age and an inspiration to us all. The workout in this book is the best for shaping, toning and losing excess body fat in record time."

—TANYA KNIGHT
Miss International and a regular on "American Gladiators"

"Gets right to the point. You don't have to dig around to find what you want—and what's more, it gets you in top shape fast!"

—LAURIE KOSZUTA, R.N., B.S.N.
Center for Hip and Knee Surgery
Mooresville, Indiana

"As a personal trainer and professional bodybuilder, I am happy to finally see a no-nonsense book that will show you how to get in shape in the shortest time possible. Not only do you burn fat and build muscle, but you speed up your metabolism too!"

—GUS STEFANIDIS
Mr. Greece

"If someone is desperate to get in shape in the quickest possible time, *The Fat-Burning Workout* is the way to go."

—LUD SHUSTERICH
World Powerlifting record holder and member of the
All Time Greats Bodybuilding Hall of Fame

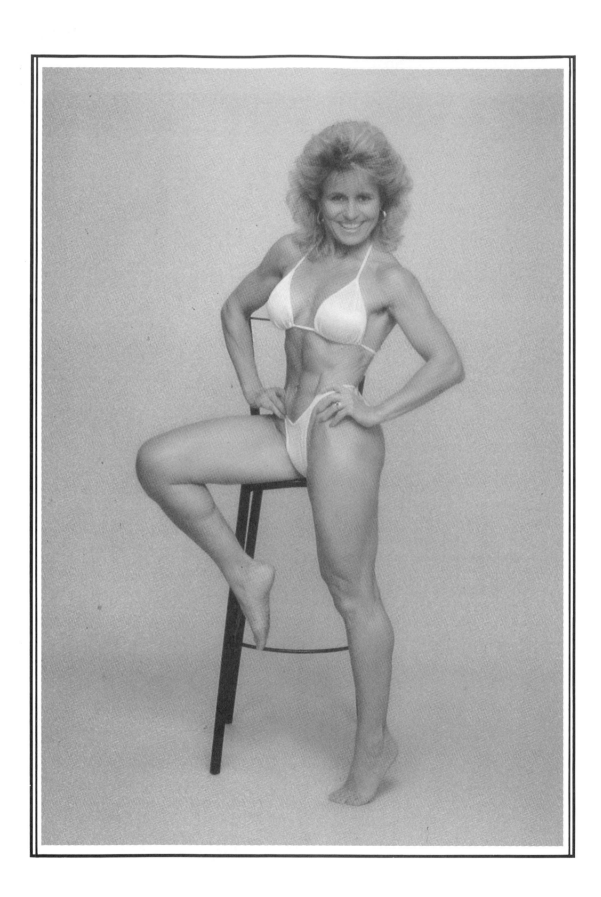

THE
FAT-BURNING
WORKOUT:

From Fat to Firm in 24 Days

Joyce L. Vedral, Ph.D.

WARNER BOOKS

A Time Warner Company

A Note from the Publisher

The ideas, procedures, and suggestions contained in this book are
not intended as a substitute for consulting with your physician.
All matters regarding your health require medical supervision.

Warner Books, Inc., 666 Fifth Avenue, New York, NY 10103

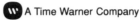 A Time Warner Company

Printed in the United States of America
First Printing: March 1991

10 9 8 7

Library of Congress Cataloging-in-Publication Data

Vedral, Joyce L.
    The fat-burning workout : from fat to firm in 24 days / Joyce L.
Vedral.
        p.   cm.
    Includes bibliographical references (p.) and index.
    ISBN 0-446-39194-8
    1. Physical fitness for women.   2. Reducing exercises.   3. Weight
training.   I. Title.
GV482.V42   1991
613.7'045—dc20

90-12487
CIP

Book design by Giorgetta Bell McRee
Cover design by Anne Twomey
Cover photo by Don Banks
Black and white photos by Don Banks
Hair and makeup by Jodi Pollutro
Cover leotard (or bathing suit) by Ziganne of Hollywood
Workout leotards by Capezio from Ballet Makers Inc.
Gym shoes by Reebok International

*To us—the women of the nineties, who know that
with good health, high energy, and total fitness,
our goals and dreams will be that much more accessible*

□

*And to Cal-a-Vie, The Ultimate Spa,
and Kent Maurer, its director, for offering women and men
an opportunity to achieve total fitness in the most luxurious
and tranquil environment possible, a spa that follows
the fitness philosophy proposed in this book!!!*

CONTENTS

ACKNOWLEDGMENTS

To Joann Davis, for guiding this project with sound judgment and generosity of time and spirit

To Colleen Kaplin, for your lively, energetic reading of the manuscript and for your timely suggestions

To Anne Twomey, for your willingness to treat this project with special care and attention

To Larry Kirshbaum, Nansey Neiman, Ling Lucas, and Ellen Herrick, for your enthusiasm and support

To Don Banks, photographer, for your creative ideas for photography and for your gifted execution of the photographs

To Joe and Betty Weider, for encouraging me in all of my fitness projects, and for providing the foundation and basis for bodybuilding in your wonderful magazines, *Shape, Muscle and Fitness, Men's Fitness,* and *Flex*

To friends and family—for being there, for loving, and for caring

To Kent Maurer—for your example of an outstanding physique and an equally delightful mind

To John Cordovano, for being there when it's important

To Cameo Kneuer, Miss National Fitness, and my friend, for your sense of humor and your steadfast presence. I love you

To Jodi Pollutro, talented hair and makeup artist, for knowing how to make a person's beauty shine

To Maria Viviane, owner of Sal-Mar Beauty Salon in Levittown, Long Island, and Jennifer Donato and Andrea Messina for your unmatchable manicures, hair, skin, and beauty care

To Gus Stefanidis, Mr. Greece and my wise confidant—a man who knows many secrets about diet and exercise

To Andy Sivert, Mr. North America, owner of Mr. America's Gym in Farmingdale, Long Island, where one can work out with the most talented people in the sport

INTRODUCTION

As a medical doctor who has specialized in diet and nutrition problems for the past five years, I have noticed that the people who gain back the weight they lost do so for one major reason: They do not have a workable exercise plan to help them maintain their weight loss.

The Fat-Burning Workout is an answer to that problem. It is an exercise plan that shapes and tones the body, increases muscle tissue, reduces fat percentage, and raises metabolism so that a person can eat more than previously and not get fat. In addition, this workout produces an aerobic effect that is highly beneficial to the heart and lungs.

Joyce Vedral provides a simple exercise plan that can be done at home in only twenty minutes. (She also offers gym alternatives and advanced plans for those who wish to go further.) In a matter of weeks, anyone following this program and doing it three to five days a week can expect to see significant improvement in muscle tone and shape, strength, posture, and energy, with the added bonus of a healthier heart and lungs and increased metabolism.

I have been recommending Vedral's books to my patients for years. They work! My patients come back and tell me they are delighted with the results. However, while Vedral's other books have been effective in shaping and toning the body, this is the first of her books that provides the exerciser with the opportunity *to burn the maximum amount of fat and at the same time shape and tone the muscles.* This is achieved through the aerobic nature of the workout. Weight training is applied in a specialized way so that maximum fat is burned.

For those of you who are not already on your own diet plan, Vedral includes an excellent low-fat diet that will result in maximum fat loss in six weeks' time. By offering a diet of 20 to 30 grams of fat daily, and by allowing the dieter to choose from an interesting variety of foods, Vedral has made eating right an exciting proposition.

For those of you who wish to get rid of a maximum of body fat in the minimum of time, and at the same time tighten, tone, and shape your body, *The Fat-Burning Workout* is the answer.

—JUDE T. BARBERA, M.D.
Assistant Clinical Professor of Surgery
Downstate Medical Center
Associate Director of Urology
Coney Island Hospital

THE
FAT-BURNING
WORKOUT

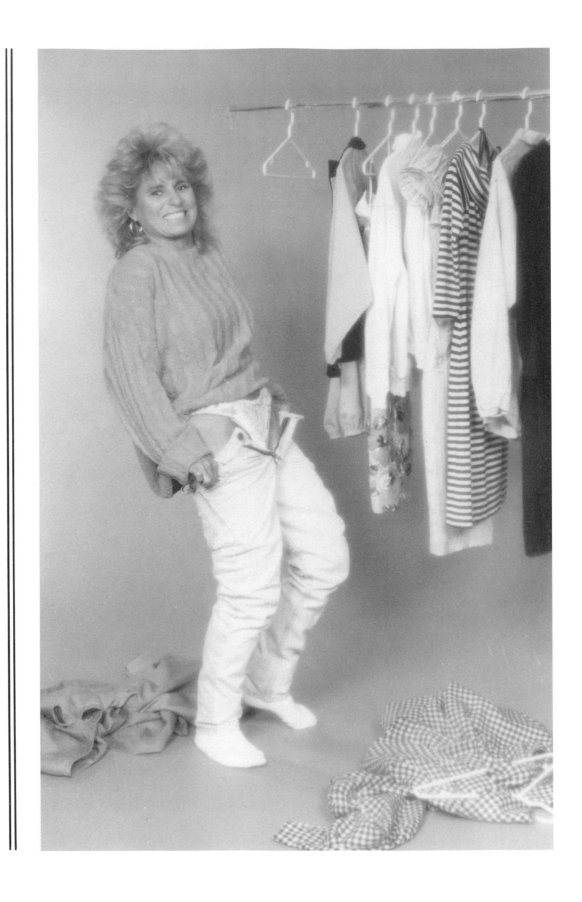

1 | HOW IT WORKS

Fat is the enemy. It causes our bodies to appear round and shapeless. It makes it impossible for us to zip up our jeans, or even get them past our hips, and what's more, it's bad for our health. Yet time and again, no matter how many times we diet it off, it returns to plague us. What is the answer to the problem? How can we get rid of the ugly fat on our bodies, once and for all, and keep it off?

If fat is the enemy, muscle is the friend. It takes up a lot less space than fat does, and what's more, it actually burns calories for us—even when we're sleeping. I'm not talking about hulking muscles—the Arnold Schwarzenegger kind. I'm referring to normal, healthy working tissue that give our bodies shape and form. So how do you get rid of fat and stock up on muscle? Health and nutrition experts are in agreement: You can't get rid of your excess body fat and keep it off unless you not only diet but exercise too. But exactly how do you diet and exercise to get and keep the fat off your potentially beautiful body?

In the following pages, you will find a workout that guarantees to rid you of those ugly rolls of fat in a matter of weeks, and to replace them with tight, toned, feminine muscles. You can choose to exercise twenty, thirty, or forty minutes, three to five times a week. *If you work out for twenty to thirty minutes four times a week, you will lose a minimum of five pounds of fat in twenty-four days, keep it off, and you'll get tight and toned at the same time, and continue to lose as much fat as you need to lose—as you follow the plan.* It's important to note that I said you will lose five pounds of fat. You see, you will probably lose about ten pounds altogether—the other five will be water, because if you haven't been eating properly, chances are, you're also retaining

2

water. As you follow the fat-burning eating plan, you'll eliminate that problem.

But the most important aspect of the fat-burning workout is that *you will keep the weight off*. The food plan and exercise program together let you lose the weight for good, and get tight, toned, and shapely at the same time.

WHY DID I WRITE THIS BOOK?

I wrote this book for all of us: for women who are impatient and even desperate, for people who have no time to play games, for people who are tired of being fooled by quick weight-loss programs that don't get you in shape. I wrote it for those who are willing to work hard for a reasonable amount of time in order to see quality results—results that last.

I wrote this book for women who want not just to be thin, but who want to have hard, sexy bodies. I wrote this book because it works, and I can't stand to know a secret that can help others without telling them about it. And most important, I wrote this book to help you get into shape, once and for all, so that you can free your mind for the other, more important issues in life.

WHAT YOU CAN EXPECT FROM THE FAT-BURNING WORKOUT

- The loss of about five pounds of fat (not water or muscle) in approximately twenty-four days
- The replacement of fat with small, shapely muscles
- A firm, sensuous, well-proportioned body
- Permanently increased metabolism so you can eat more without getting fat
- A healthier outlook on food and eating—and a specific diet plan
- Lifetime maintenance in the shape you want to be in
- A healthier heart and greater lung capacity
- More energy
- Improved posture
- Increased self-confidence

HOW WAS THIS PROGRAM DISCOVERED?

When working out in the gym, I often noticed champion bodybuilders using giant sets, the training method described in this book. Only, at the time I didn't know why. After years of interviewing bodybuilders for articles on health and fitness magazines, I discovered that they had one reason and one reason alone for using this method. That reason was to burn fat while making their muscles harder at the same time.

"Now, isn't this the goal of every woman," I thought, "to get rid of fat and to tighten and tone her body?" But because of my busy schedule, I did nothing about my discovery at the time . . . until I got myself in trouble one winter by gaining ten pounds and then was asked to do an unexpected photo shoot in just three and a half weeks. Motivated to try a new plan of action, I put together a workout based upon the giant set, which I'll describe in a moment. Only I modified it according to my needs. I created my own version of the technique, using much lighter weights and exercises more appropriate to a woman's goals. Amazingly, I got rid of five pounds of fat in twenty-four days. I also lost three pounds of water. (The body gives up a pound to a pound and a half of fat per week, not much more, so I assume the rest was water. It certainly wasn't muscle. I had *gained* muscle.) I was able to live with the remaining two extra pounds because of the great shape I was in, although after another two weeks of following this plan, I lost them, too!

After that, I enlisted countless women in my experiment and found that a program of modified giant sets is the most effective method I've ever seen to get rid of fat and tighten and tone the body in record time. It is intense, but it works fast, and the results last.

WHY WHAT YOU'VE TRIED HASN'T WORKED

The most common methods of getting rid of fat are not efficient. Starvation diets—those that require you to consume less than 1,000 calories per day—help you to lose weight, but much of what you lose will be water, some of it will be muscle, and only a little bit of it will be fat. The problem with these diets is that you end up flabby anyway, and you're still ashamed of your body in a bathing suit or in the nude. And what's worse, you quickly gain the weight back. The body is a survival system, and after you have starved it, it waits for the

4

moment you are off guard and then compels you to eat and eat and eat—until it has a reserve of fat stored up for the next time it's threatened with starvation.

So the starvation diet system is a vicious circle. It works only for a week or two —you'll be very temporarily thinner. Then you'll gain the weight back—and you'll end up fatter than you were in the first place. That's because when you starve yourself, you lose one pound of muscle for every three pounds of fat you lose. When you gain the weight back, it all comes back as fat. The only way to gain muscle is to work for it—as described in this program, for example.

In addition, starvation diets cause your overall metabolism to slow down, so that once you stop dieting, you end up gaining weight even if you don't overeat.

The other most commonly used method of getting rid of fat is aerobic activity such as running, bicycling, rope-jumping, and aerobic dancing. While these things do help to burn quite a bit of fat, that's basically all they do. They don't reshape your sagging body parts. They don't give you a flat stomach, perfectly shaped thighs, firm buttocks, an uplifted chest, shapely arms, and so on. Aerobic activities in and of themselves can do just so much for you. They can help to keep your heart and lungs healthy, and they can help you to burn some overall body fat, but to really shape up takes something more.

WHAT DOES WORK?

What you need is a program that can burn fat and at the same time tighten, tone, and shape muscles. What you need is *The Fat-Burning Workout*. The workout in chapters 6 and 7, coupled with the eating plan in chapter 8, will get you to your goal in a matter of weeks. This program is designed for women who mean business. It's a one-shot exercise plan that burns the maximum of fat while at the same time it sculpts petite muscles on nine parts of the body: your biceps, chest, shoulders, triceps, back, thighs, buttocks, abdominals, and calves. What you end up with is not only a lean, shapely body, but one that is well proportioned and esthetically appealing —a body that is composed of lean tissue rather than fat—a body that can now consume more calories than before without gaining weight.

Why build muscle? Because muscle is the only body material that is active rather than passive. Muscles burn calories merely by existing. Fat just lies there on your body, stagnant. The more muscle tissue you have on your body, the faster your body burns calories.

Simply put, when you increase the amount of muscle you have, your resting metabolic rate goes up. So where you used to burn, say, 80 calories an hour just sitting in a chair thinking, you now burn between 100 and 120 calories per hour doing the same thing. The same higher rate of calorie burning follows you through the day and night, so that no matter what you are doing, whether walking, running, talking, or even sleeping, you are burning more calories than you would if your body were composed of less muscle and more fat. Once you have increased the muscle tissue on your body and reduced the fat, you can eat more than you used to eat—without getting fat. Have you noticed that men seem to be able to eat so much more than women without getting fat? That's because on the average men have a much greater muscle mass than do women. And women, on average, have a higher proportion of fat.

YOU CAN INCREASE MUSCLE TISSUE WITHOUT GETTING BIG MUSCLES

As a woman, the last thing you want to do is put big, bulky muscles on your body. Chances are you've seen female bodybuilders in magazines or on television and thought to yourself, "Who wants to look like that?"

You can put your mind at ease. The kind of muscles you will build with the Fat-Burning Workout are small, firm, well-defined muscles—the sensuous, shapely kind, not the masculine, bulky kind.

In fact, there's a built-in guarantee in this program that you won't get big muscles, because you will be exercising with very light weights. I am friends with many champion female bodybuilders, and I know what they must do in order to get those large muscles: They have to spend at least twelve hours a week working out with very heavy weights—up to 250 pounds for some body parts. So don't worry. If you follow this program, it can't happen to you.

ALL THIS AND AEROBICS, TOO?

Most fitness experts have long considered it impossible to burn fat aerobically and build firm and shapely muscles at the same time. But bodybuilders have known the secret to achieving these goals simultaneously for years: the giant set. They use it just before contests, when they want to perfect the quality of their muscles without adding any significant size. The giant set entails exercising a muscle intensely. The exerciser does one set each of three different exercises for a body part without resting. Bodybuilders use rather heavy weights, even with this grueling routine.

6

The Fat-Burning Workout modifies the giant set to use lighter weights so you can work even faster. Working fast allows you to burn the maximum amount of fat by maintaining a heart rate of at least 70 percent of your capacity for twenty minutes or more. And using lighter weights ensures that you build only small, shapely muscles. The body will only build large muscles if you force it to do so by making it lift heavier and heavier weights.

Weight training has traditionally been considered an anaerobic activity, an activity that cannot be supported by the body's natural oxygen supply, so that frequent rest periods are needed. When you lift heavy weights, your body depends upon quick bursts of energy and significant rests. The rests are necessary to replenish the body's oxygen. Although the Fat-Burning Workout uses weights, it is an aerobic activity. Because the weights used are so light, you can work at a steady pace and use your body's natural, steady flow of oxygen. You do not have to take lengthy rests to replenish your supply.

HOW DOES THIS WORKOUT COMPARE TO REGULAR WEIGHT TRAINING?

What then is the difference between the Fat-Burning Workout and other weight training programs, including programs laid out in my other books, *Now or Never*, *Perfect Parts*, and *Hard Bodies*?

In regular weight training programs the individual performs three to five exercises per body part—just as in this program. But there is a big difference with the Fat-Burning Workout: rest times.

In a regular workout system—like the one in *Now or Never*, for example—one performs the first chest exercise, the bench press, by doing the first set of fifteen repetitions, resting for thirty seconds, doing ten repetitions, resting for thirty seconds, and then doing a final set of eight repetitions and resting for another thirty seconds before proceeding to the next chest exercise. In the Fat-Burning Workout giant set, the individual does the first set of all three to five chest exercises (depending on the plan chosen) without resting. Then—and only then—is a rest allowed, but it is a short rest of only ten to fifteen seconds. The individual then does the second set of all three to five exercises, takes another short rest, and finally, completes the last set.

ISN'T THIS JUST LIKE CIRCUIT TRAINING?

It sounds much like circuit training, but it isn't. Circuit training requires that you do one exercise per body part for about a minute before moving on to the next body part. However, the Fat-Burning Workout, like champion bodybuilders, uses the principle of muscle isolation. It demands that you do at least *three exercises for one body part* before moving on to the next body part.

As any professional bodybuilder will tell you, circuit training can never significantly reshape body parts. Why? It does not ask you to do enough exercises for each body part in sequence to make a difference. For example, in circuit training, you are asked to do one exercise for, say, your chest, and then you must move to an exercise for another body part, say your shoulders, and then to another and so on. While some fat is burned in this manner, little is accomplished in the area of muscle shaping. The people who invented circuit training were not champion bodybuilders. They were manufacturers of gym machinery, and their goal was to sell more gym equipment.

Don't misunderstand. I'm not saying that circuit training is useless. It has its purpose. You can use it to burn some calories, to get quick total-body stimulation, and to help condition your heart and lungs. But if you're hoping that circuit training will reshape your body, you're in for a big disappointment, as those of you who have tried it already know.

The full Fat-Burning Workout technique is simple to understand and fully spelled out in chapter 5. For now, keep in mind that this workout is much more intense than a regular body-building workout—but it is easier to do because you are lifting much lighter weights. Also, because of its intensity, you work faster, so you get finished faster.

In regular weight training systems such as described in *Now or Never*, *Hard Bodies*, and *Perfect Parts*, you are expected to go as heavy as you can for each set. (You might use fifteen-pound dumbbells for your first bench press set, twenty for your second set, and twenty-five for your third.) As a result, you build muscle mass—more than some women like. The Fat-Burning Workout requires no such thing. In fact, you are not allowed to go heavy at all. You must use sets of three-, five-, and ten-pound dumbbells (or slightly heavier weights if you have already been lifting weights for a while). The end result: you burn fat due to the steady pace and speed, and your entire body is firmed and attractively shaped because the exercises resculpt the muscles in each of your nine body parts.

HOW DOES THIS PROGRAM COMPARE TO THE 12-MINUTE TOTAL-BODY WORKOUT?

My 12-Minute Total-Body Workout requires that the individual substitute weight for self-imposed pressure—"dynamic tension" and isometric pressure. The person works for twelve minutes using only three-pound dumbbells and, by the end of the week, has exercised the entire body twice and the buttocks and abdominals three times. The workout is very intense and tightens and tones the muscles. However, while this workout does in and of itself help the exerciser to exerciser to burn quite a bit of fat, in order to obtain an aerobic workout, those following the workout must do *an additional* twenty minutes of aerobic activity.

In the Fat-Burning Workout, extra aerobics are suggested for those who wish to speed up their progress or burn additional fat, or for those who enjoy aerobic activities. However, they are not required, because the Fat-Burning Workout is in and of itself an aerobic exercise, in addition to being a body-shaping activity.

HOW DOES THIS WORKOUT COMPARE TO GENERAL SPORTS?

No sport can help to reshape one's entire body into near perfect symmetry. If anything, a sport can only affect the body parts that are directly involved with that sport. For example, tennis, paddleball, and racquetball players have lovely, muscular forearms. Gymnasts, swimmers, and judo experts have highly developed backs and shoulders. Soccer players, ballet dancers, and horseback riders have gorgeous legs. And so on.

It is foolish to depend upon your sport to reshape your body. At its best, your sport can help to test your strength, flexibility, endurance, and skill and can assist you in burning some calories. It can also put you in a great mood. Because these are significant benefits, I recommend that you continue to participate in your favorite sport, but do that in addition to this workout.

HOW MUCH TIME WILL YOU HAVE TO INVEST?

The regular Fat-Burning Workout requires only three to five weekly sessions of twenty minutes each. Can you spare that much time? I'm sure you can. Give up just one telephone conversation and you'll have your twenty minutes. Or you can relinquish reading the paper. There are so many places you can find twenty minutes to spare in those three to five days in your week.

If you want to get in shape even faster, you may choose the Intensity Fat-Burning Program. This program takes thirty minutes, three to five times a week. If you really want to go wild, you can choose the Insanity Fat-Burning Program and invest forty minutes three to five times a week. It's your choice. But no matter which program you choose, you will see significant results in twenty-four days, and you will probably get to your goal in less than six weeks, depending upon the shape you are in now. (See chapter 2 for details.)

A SPECIAL PROMISE TO THOSE OF YOU WHO ARE VERY, VERY FAT

If you are fifty pounds overweight, I'll get you into shape in six months. If you are a hundred pounds overweight, I'll get you in shape in a year. Too long? Not really. Six months . . . twelve months. They pass quickly in any event. And when they're over you will either be in the same shape, worse shape, or better shape.

Why not make it better shape? Why not give this program a try? And I'll tell you what. I won't abandon you either. You can write to me as you go along, and if you enclose a stamped, self-addressed envelope, I promise to answer you and to help you along.

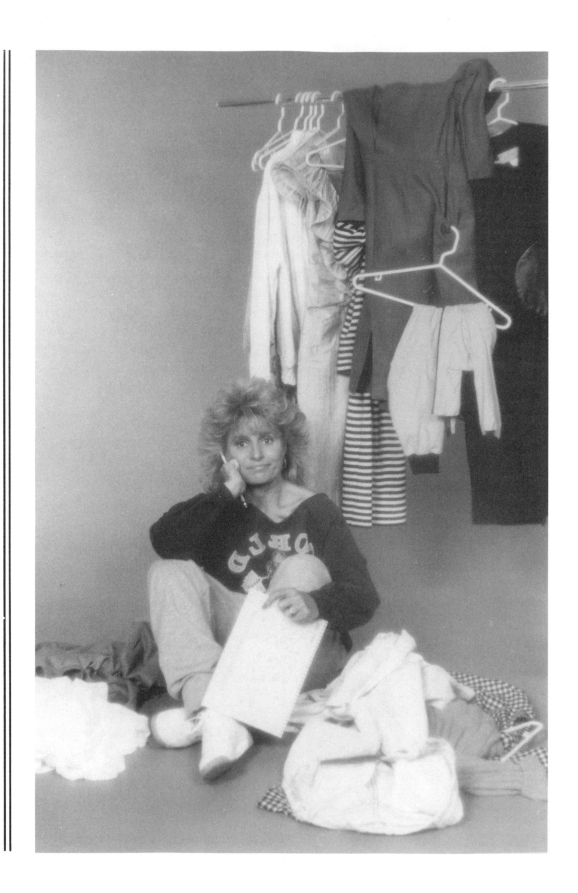

2 | WHERE ARE YOU NOW?

Y ou want to get rid of the fat *now*. You wish there were a short-cut—one that would get you to your goal in a matter of days or even hours. Well, while I can't promise you such miracles as that, I can promise you that if you follow this program rigorously, you will see significant results in three weeks, and if you are from ten to fifteen pounds overweight, you'll lose those excess pounds in about six weeks.

The exact rate of your progress will depend upon two things: your present condition and the amount of time you're willing to invest in the program. First, let's talk about your present condition.

WEIGHT VERSUS BEING IN SHAPE

Right now I weigh one hundred and twenty-three pounds. I'm exactly five feet tall, and I'm in great shape. I'm a little heavier than I like to be for photo shoots and television shows (my ideal weight is 115) but I still look good in a bikini. I do have some extra body fat, but put me next to a woman my height and the same weight who doesn't work out and she will look like a blimp next to me. Why?

She will have a lot more fat on her body than I do. My weight is muscle

12   weight, not fat weight. Muscle is condensed material, so it weighs more than fat but takes up less space.

Think of it this way: Inch for inch, muscle weighs more than fat. Muscle is to fat as lead is to feathers. An inch of lead weighs more than an inch of feathers, right? A feather-filled pillow looks fatter than a square inch of lead, but it may weigh the same. Get the picture?

Of course, the above example is somewhat exaggerated. Muscle really weighs only about two and a half times as much as fat does. But the point is clear. The scale is not always the best gauge to use when trying to get in shape—especially if your goal is to gain muscle tone and to get rid of the enemy—fat.

HOW CAN YOU TELL IF YOU'RE FAT

Chances are, if you think you're fat you are. Even if you're not overweight you can be fat. There are two kinds of fat—fat fat and skinny fat. Fat fat is overweight and fat. If you are fat fat, you can clearly see a roll of lard on your lower belly, lumps of fat on your hips, and rows of bunched up fat (commonly called cellulite) on your thighs. You will also notice that your buttocks seem to have taken over a larger proportion of your body, invading the area of your lower back and thighs.

If you are skinny fat, on the other hand, you probably don't have rolls of lard anywhere (except maybe a very small roll on your lower belly), but you are still fat. How do you know? You are basically soft to the touch—too soft. For example, if you poke your finger into your thigh or your arm, your finger goes into your flesh more deeply than it should. In fact, it feels as if your finger could go right through your arm, to the bone. This happens because you are touching the soft, spongy fat that is right under your skin, rather than the firm, taut muscle that should be there—and that will be there after you use the Fat-Burning Workout for a while. In short, if you are a skinny fat, you are not overweight, but your body is composed of too much fatty tissue and not enough muscle tissue. If you're a skinny fat, you will not lose weight on this program, you'll just get in shape.

IT'S WHAT YOU SEE IN THE MIRROR THAT COUNTS

You don't have to worry about height-weight charts if you don't want to. Because of the above truths, height-weight charts are not always accurate. And even if they were accurate, who cares? It's what you see in the mirror that counts anyway, right? So no matter what you weigh now, you needn't bother to weigh yourself at all as you follow this workout. Just look in the mirror and see what is happening as you go along. The mirror doesn't lie or fool you. Sometimes the scale does (water fluctuation, recent elimination, etc.).

FOR THOSE OF YOU WHO ARE NOT SO DARING

The fact is, most people are not so daring as to just diet and follow a workout program without getting on a scale. Even if they see the results in the mirror, they want to see those results also registered on the scale. In addition, most people are too curious not to get on the scale and at least see what's happening. Finally, most people are just too conditioned to using the scale as a measuring device to stop "cold turkey" and replace the scale with the mirror.

For this reason, I will help those of you who want to think in terms of scale weight to do so realistically, in the hope that as you approach being in near-perfect shape, you will see for yourself that the scale is not as important as the mirror. With this in mind, let us begin our discussion on height and weight.

BONE STRUCTURE PLAYS A ROLE

Your overall bone structure refers to your frame and your height combined—in other words, your skeleton. It determines the basic silhouette of your body without excess fat. Your frame refers to the size of your bones and the way they are placed, irrespective of your height.

We cannot alter our bone structure by dieting. When it comes to being able to carry weight without looking fat, taller, larger-framed women are luckier than shorter, smaller-framed women, because the weight is spread out over a larger area. If a short, small-framed woman weighed as much as a tall, large-framed woman, she would look fat. So short, small-framed women have to eat less than their larger female counterparts in order to stay in shape.

YOU CAN GET INTO SHAPE NO MATTER WHAT YOUR BONE STRUCTURE

If you want to follow this program and get into the best possible shape for you, all you have to do is stick with it until you reach your goal. What difference does it make if you're short or tall, big boned or small boned? The only difference is how hard you have to work to get and stay in shape.

I'm not lucky. I'm short, and I have a medium frame. In addition, I come from a Russian family. It was always a tradition in my grandmother's house to have at least four meat dishes on the table at dinner, not to mention all kinds of greasy cabbage dishes. What's more, if anyone got up from the table with even a hint of alacrity, my grandmother would become highly insulted. If you didn't stuff yourself to the fullest possible extent, in her mind that meant you didn't really like her cooking.

It is probably for this reason that my grandmother and many of her friends looked as if they were large squares on wheels as they moved about from place to place. I can still see my grandmother (who was just under five feet) gliding around in her long green coat, her little feet sticking out from the bottom of the coat and a "babushka" (kerchief) on her head. It really looked as if she were rolling along, not walking.

If I had not been careful, I would by now be well on my way to looking like my grandmother. In fact, for a while I was on that exact trail. But, thank God, I ran into professional bodybuilders who taught me the right way to get in shape and stay there. I've been sharing my knowledge with my readers ever since, in *Now or Never*, *The Twelve-Minute Total-Body Workout*, *Perfect Parts*, and *Hard Bodies*.

IF I CAN DO IT, SO CAN YOU

Sometimes I have to laugh at myself. Even though I don't have the ideal figure (I'm not tall, and let's face it, I do have big hips) (look at my back anatomy photograph, p. 46) I dare to feature myself on the cover and in inside photos of exercise books. Why do I do this? I do it because I know that there are thousands of other women out there, just like me, who don't have, and never will have, the potential to be long-legged models. I want to encourage these women to get into the best shape they possibly can. And I also want to encourage the women who are out of shape and who do have the potential to have classical model figures. To those women, I want to say in all sincerity, "You can look even better than I do."

You might be thinking, "Who is she kidding? She looks great. She could win a bathing beauty contest." No. I never could and I never will win such a contest. In fact, I did enter a bathing beauty contest twice, and both times I came in close to last place. Why? They seemed to be looking for tall, young, long-legged beauties—not a five-foot-tall woman who had long since said good-bye to thirty!

A SAMPLE HEIGHT AND WEIGHT CHART

After studying various height-weight charts, I found that the Metropolitan Life Insurance Company chart, published in 1983, is the most appropriate one for my purposes. As you look at the chart, first determine your frame. Then you will be able to see whether or not you are within the range of weight suggested for your height.

When calculating, remember that the chart allows for three pounds of clothing and one-inch heels, so if you are like most women and measure your height in bare feet and weigh yourself in the nude, you must look at the chart column for a woman one inch taller than you. In addition, you must subtract three pounds from the chart weight designated for you. Finally, since you are at this point not very muscular, you should *not* really weigh the maximum allowed in your column. At most you should weigh only six pounds more than the minimum. It is only later, after you have put on some muscle, that your weight should be allowed to reach the maximum for your column without your being considered overweight, or as I should say overfat! The reason for this extra allowance of weight later is due to the fact that muscle tissue weighs more than fat.

Before you can use the chart efficiently, you will have to determine your frame. You will need a partner for this.

Extend your arm and bend your forearm upward at a 90-degree angle. Turn the inside of your wrist toward your body, and extend your fingers straight out. Place the thumb and index fingers of your other hand on the bones that protrude on either side of your elbow. Have your partner take a ruler and measure the space between your fingers. (If you try to do this yourself, by the time you move your fingers away from your elbow area, you will have probably moved your fingers and lost the measurement. It's better, for the sake of accuracy, to use a partner.)

After you have gotten the measurement, compare it to those listed on the frame determination table here, which gives the measurements for medium-framed women. If your measurements fall within the range of the table, you are medium-framed. If they fall below those given in the table, you are a small-framed woman, and if they are higher, you are a large-framed woman.

MEDIUM FRAME DETERMINATION TABLE

Height in 1″ Heels	Space Between Elbow Bones
4′ 10″–5′ 3″	2¼″–2½″
5′ 4″–5′ 11″	2⅜″–2⅝″
6′ 0″–	2½″–2¾″

Now you are ready to find your ideal weight range on the height-weight chart.

HEIGHT-WEIGHT CHART

Height Feet	Height Inches	Small Frame	Medium Frame	Large Frame
4	10	102–111	109–121	118–131
4	11	103–113	111–123	120–134
5	0	104–115	113–126	122–137
5	1	106–118	115–129	125–140
5	2	108–121	118–132	128–143
5	3	111–124	121–135	131–147
5	4	114–127	124–138	134–151
5	5	117–130	127–141	137–156
5	6	120–133	130–144	140–159
5	7	123–136	133–147	143–163
5	8	126–139	136–150	146–167
5	9	129–142	139–153	149–170
5	10	132–145	142–156	152–173
5	11	135–148	145–159	155–176
6	0	138–151	148–162	158–179

As you will notice, there is quite a large weight-range allowance. As discussed above, we are going to shorten this range. Here's how. To calculate whether or not you're overweight, find yourself on the chart and add six pounds to the lowest allowed weight. For example, if you are medium framed and five feet four inches (you must look at the 5' 5" column, remembering that the chart allows for one inch heels), your lowest range is 127. However, remember that the chart has allowed for three pounds of clothing, so if you weigh yourself in the nude, you must deduct three additional pounds. This brings you to 124 for your lowest weight. The regular chart would allow you twelve pounds beyond that for your highest acceptable weight. That is too high, especially since you do not have a lot of muscle on your body. I allow you only six pounds higher. In this case, that brings you to 130. So if you are a woman who is five feet four inches tall and have a medium frame, every pound over 130 is overweight. Thus, if you weigh 140 pounds, you can consider yourself to be ten pounds overweight, and in the first category discussed below. Determine which category you belong to and read that section.

ONE TO FIFTEEN POUNDS OVERWEIGHT

If you are not more than one to fifteen pounds overweight, I can practically guarantee that if you follow the regular workout in this book, you will reach your goal in six weeks' time—maybe sooner. You will lose eight to ten pounds of solid lard, plus about five pounds of excess water—and if you follow the maintenance plan discussed in chapter 10, you'll keep it off. Your body will become muscular, shapely, and well-defined.

If in six weeks your scale weight does not go down the full ten pounds, don't worry about it. Since muscle weighs more than fat, chances are your fat weight has gone down while your muscle weight has gone up. The proportion of each in your body has changed, and that was your goal to begin with. You have added muscle while subtracting fat, so your weight may not go down as much as it would have had you not gained muscle. However, because muscle is more condensed than fat, you will still be smaller in size—you will probably have gone down at least two dress sizes. Here's where you start realizing that it's not what you see on the scale that counts, but what you see in the mirror. Muscular people are not all that concerned with the scale, and soon you will realize that you too can free yourself of the bondage to the scale. You have a new measuring device to account to. The mirror.

SIXTEEN TO THIRTY POUNDS OVERWEIGHT

If you are around thirty pounds overweight, it will take you about fifteen weeks to lose the weight, assuming that some of your weight is water weight. It is impossible for the body to lose much more than a pound and a half to two pounds of fat a week. (The average amount is usually a pound to a pound and a half of actual fat.) Anything in excess of that is usually water. If you try to lose weight faster by starving yourself, you will lose muscle tissue along with the fat. Then, instead of feeling firm and toned when you reach your goal, you will feel flabby and soft.

You may lose more than thirty pounds in twelve weeks, however, if some of your excess weight is water bloat. If this happens, you are lucky. You will reach your weight goal faster.

Don't be discouraged if your body seems to come to a standstill once you are within a few pounds of your goal. The closer you get to your goal, the more difficult it is to lose weight. Remember, the body is not vain. It is a survival system and always likes to keep a few pounds of fat stored up for the future.

But chances are you won't actually have to lose the thirty pounds you thought you had to lose. Why? Because muscle weighs more than fat, and you are gaining muscle while losing fat. Once you are in shape, you may be able to weigh the maximum indicated on the chart and be in perfect shape.

Before I started working out, I had to weigh 112 pounds to look as "thin" as I do now at 123 pounds. In addition, I look better now because I have a better shape and my body is tight and toned.

THIRTY-ONE TO FIFTY POUNDS OVERWEIGHT

If you are fifty pounds overweight, don't despair. It will just take you a little longer to get in shape—about twenty-five weeks.

The good news is that you've got a good chance of losing the full two pounds maximum of fat each week, because the fatter you are, the more willing your body is to give up fat. And chances are you are holding a lot of excess water, too. People who are extremely overweight tend to retain more water than those who are not so overweight. As you follow the Fat-Burning Workout and Eating

Plan, you will also lose the excess water. So you might end up losing an average of more than two pounds a week in the beginning, because some of it will be water. This will encourage you to keep going in the beginning, when you need the encouragement most.

If you lose two pounds of fat a week, in twelve weeks you will have lost twenty-four pounds of pure fat. In addition, if you lose eight pounds of water, you will have lost thirty pounds in the first twelve weeks. That would bring you to twenty pounds away from your goal. Amazingly, even at that weight, you will look great. Better than you ever did before at that weight. Why? Because, as noted above, your body composition will have shifted. Your body will now be composed of more muscle, which is denser and weighs more, and less fat, which is more spread out but weighs less. The end result will be that you look much slimmer than you did at this same weight before. In fact, you may find that instead of having to lose another twenty pounds, you only have to lose another ten.

MORE THAN FIFTY POUNDS OVERWEIGHT

If you are fifty or more pounds overweight, it's not a good idea to embark on any weight-loss or shape-up plan without first consulting your doctor—or even better, a doctor who specializes in diet and nutrition. Show this program to your doctor, and allow him or her to adjust it, if need be, to your specific medical needs.

If the doctor agrees, and you follow this shape-up plan, you can expect to lose an average of two pounds a week for the first three months (a combination of water and fat weight) and an average of about a pound and a half a week (this will be pure fat) after that. Assuming you are a hundred pounds overweight to begin with, this will bring you to a weight loss of about eighty-four pounds in a year's time. Now you will only have sixteen pounds more to lose, but chances are, since you will have increased the amount of your muscle tissue while decreasing body fat, your weight will no longer mean you are overweight. A look in the mirror may confirm that you are at your goal or that you only have a few more pounds to lose.

SPEEDING UP THE PROCESS WITH THE INTENSITY AND INSANITY PLANS

The preceding weight-loss projections are based upon the regular fat-burning workout plan, employed four times a week. If you wish to speed up your progress, you may choose to work with the Intensity or Insanity plans, or you may choose to work five times a week instead of four times a week. (See chapter 5 for a discussion of the three workout plans.)

For those of you who can only work out three times a week, if you use the Intensity or Insanity plan, chances are you will make the same progress as those who work out four days a week and use the regular plan. But the quickest way to get in shape is to use the Insanity plan five days a week. (See chapter 9 for other ways to speed up your progress.)

WHAT DOES AGE HAVE TO DO WITH IT?

As you get older, it takes you a little longer to lose weight because your metabolism slows down due to muscle atrophy. We lose a tiny fraction of muscle tissue each year after thirty. Most experts believe that this is due to decreased physical activity. However, if you build up your body's muscle, your metabolism will speed up, no matter what your age. In fact, as I got older, my metabolism increased rather than slowed down. Why? Because by conscious effort I put back on the muscle that was being atrophied—and then some. So now I burn more calories per hour than I did when I was thirty—and you can, too.

There is another factor that slows older people down when it comes to getting in shape. Younger people seem to build muscle more quickly and heal more quickly than do older people. Young muscles seem to respond more quickly to change and challenge than do old muscles. For this reason, when it comes to muscle-shaping, you can expect to tighten and tone your body according to the average schedule I've indicated if you are around thirty-five years old. If you are younger than that, your body will respond more quickly. If you are older than that, your body will respond a little more slowly. How much more quickly or slowly? That's difficult to predict. A lot depends on your genetics. But the difference will not be more than a few weeks longer or shorter than I've described, no matter what your age. In this respect, I am lucky. I can get in shape in less than six weeks, using the Insanity plan five times a week if I'm ten pounds overweight—and I'm forty-seven years old.

CAN YOU STOP WORKING OUT ONCE YOU GET IN SHAPE?

Of course not. But you don't necessarily have to follow this grueling routine for the rest of your life. See chapter 10 for a variety of choices for lifetime maintenance.

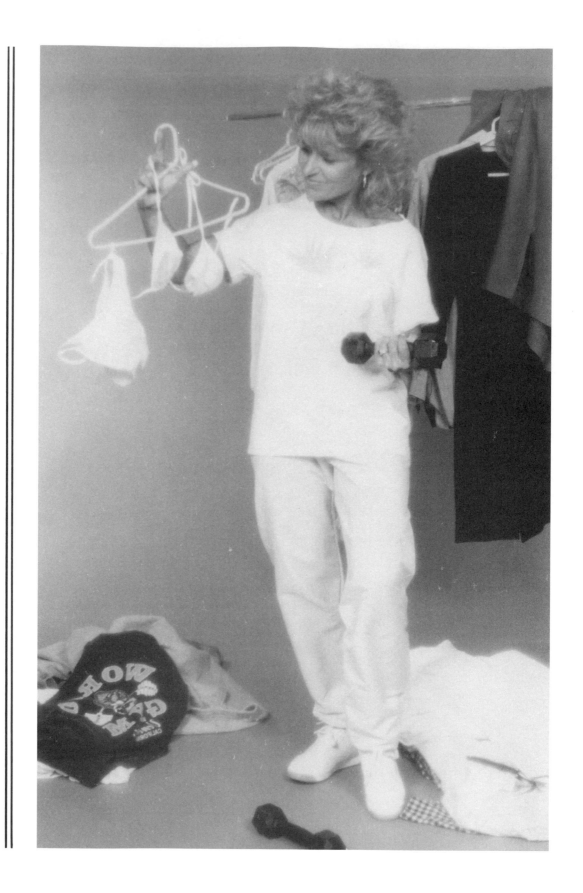

3 | THE MENTAL WORKOUT

First the desire, then the deed. Every accomplishment begins with a thought—a desire. How badly do you want to lose that unsightly fat that covers your potentially curvaceous body? Can you picture yourself strutting down the beach in a bathing suit as you sense the admiration of others? Can you imagine how wonderful it will be not to have to hide your body, no matter what the situation?

The first step to accomplishing your goal is desire. You can increase your desire by imagining the way you will feel ahead of time. Let your mind run free. See yourself slim, in shape, and happy. Then relax and realize that it is going to happen this time, because finally, you really want it.

SO WHAT IF YOU FAILED BEFORE!

Perhaps the most important thing you can do to help yourself get in shape is to forgive yourself for past failures. Self-reproach only serves to drain your energy.

If you've failed to get in shape many times in the past, it's probably because you were knocking on the wrong doors. It's like looking for the right job. People often pound the pavement for months, and have to endure countless rejections before they finally hit upon the job that is perfect for them. What would happen if they just quit trying? They would end up on public assistance—permanently.

Fortunately, this is not what happens in most cases. In fact, most people have a fighting spirit, even if it does take some time for them to get their second wind. In fact, there's something buried deep down within every human being that whispers a message of hope, even in the moments of darkest despair. "Try again. Maybe this time it will work." So that's what you're doing now. You're trying again. And this time, *it will work*.

Another reason you may have failed in the past is that perhaps you were not really ready to get in shape at the time. Maybe there were other, more pressing things on your mind. Now, for some reason, you are ready, and you know it. The fact that you're reading this book and not one of those miracle-plan books that promises to get you in shape by some special machine or in only a week's time is a good sign. The fact is, you're ready to pay a realistic price for something you desire with a passion.

Finally, you might have failed in the past because you were asked to do the impossible. Who wouldn't rebel against starving oneself half to death or eating tasteless, unappealing food? And who wouldn't quit a fitness regimen that required hours of exhausting exercise? Fortunately, this plan allows you to eat delicious, nutritious foods, and eventually allows you to have any food you like, no matter how "naughty" it is. It also asks you to work out for a minimum of three twenty-minute sessions a week, and a maximum of five forty-minute sessions a week. Somewhere within this plan, there's a realistic pace for you.

PREPARING YOUR MIND FOR THE WORKOUT

Before you start working out, it's important to give yourself time to prepare mentally for what you will be doing. In other words, you need to "psych" yourself before you start the program. In order to do this, it's important that you read this book from cover to cover before ever picking up a weight.

The next thing you'll want to do is give yourself an official "start date." For example, you may decide to start one week from today. Between now and your start date, your goal will be to become excited about the prospect of working out. A few simple actions will help with this process.

As you read the book, read with a pen in your hand and underline ideas that strike you as important. You may also want to make comments in the margin, such as "That's the way I feel," or "Exactly," and so on. If you do this, you will become an active rather than a passive reader, and your chances of permanently absorbing not only the content but also the spirit of the book will be greatly increased.

While you are reading the book, start looking around for your equipment: a set each of three-, five-, and ten-pound dumbbells and a flat exercise bench that can be raised to an incline. You can purchase these items in any sporting goods store or they can be ordered directly from me. (See page 205 for information.)

Then, once your equipment is in the house, don't hide it away. Leave it out where you can see it. Place the dumbbells in your bedroom or den. Line the bench up against the wall. (Even the smallest apartment can accommodate the narrow exercise bench.) Allow the workout equipment to become a symbol of life and growth. Be happy every time you catch a glimpse of it.

If you're planning to work out in a gym, look around for the appropriate facility. If you're already a member of a health club but haven't been going, begin to picture yourself doing this workout in your fitness center. Recall where the dumbbells and benches are kept. Imagine yourself doing the alternate gym exercises. But remember, once you go to the gym, don't let anyone talk you into using a different program. I can't vouch for a program your gym may give you, whereas I can guarantee the results of this one.

IF YOU STILL HAVE SERIOUS DOUBTS THAT YOU CAN SUCCEED

For those of you who are by nature skeptical, I have good news. Even if you don't really believe this program will work, it will anyway—as long as you follow it exactly. Just say to yourself, "I don't have to believe it. I just have to do it." Then do it.

Do it by an act of sheer will. Whenever the thought comes to you, "You're wasting your time, you fool," just look at that thought, acknowledge it, and think, "That's nice. But I'm going to do it anyway." By taking action in spite of your doubts, you will be doing your part. The program will take care of the rest. You'll begin to see results in spite of yourself. And don't let anyone discourage you. A friend of mine did this workout in her local gym. The first day, the owner of the gym laughed at her. She was 30 pounds overweight and out of shape. "You can't do that workout," he said. "It's too advanced for you." Three months later she did a photo shoot for a magazine and people in the gym were asking for her advice.

POSITIVE THINKING CAN HELP YOU GET TO YOUR GOAL FASTER

No matter what the challenge facing you, it's always more productive to face it with optimism rather than pessimism. This fact can be demonstrated most readily in the area of surgery. A recent study has demonstrated that people who have a positive outlook on the outcome of surgery consistently fare better than those who have a negative outlook, all other things being equal. In fact, in their book *Healthy Pleasures*, Robert Ornstein and David Sobel note that the large majority of patients who are optimistic have fewer complications, a shorter hospital stay, and a shorter recovery time.

This does not surprise me one bit. It is virtually impossible to ignore the fact that mental attitude counts when it comes to success at any undertaking. Fifty years ago, original thinkers such as Norman Vincent Peale, Dale Carnegie, and Maxwell Maltz were expounding this idea. They were ahead of their time. Today, we have proof positive of such truths. Dr. Bernie Siegel, Dr. Joan Borysenko, Dr. Robert Ornstein, Norman Cousins and a host of others have now offered case studies that clearly demonstrate that the mind plays a major role in overcoming seemingly insurmountable obstacles (see the bibliography).

With this in mind, I encourage you to cooperate with yourself by inviting your mind to assist you in achieving your goal. Here are some time-tested ways to speed up, even double, your progress.

DECIDE WHAT YOU WANT TO LOOK LIKE AND VISUALIZE YOUR BODY EVOLVING INTO THAT IMAGE

Get a realistic picture in your mind of the shape you want to be in. When I say realistic, I'm not kidding. There's no sense in imagining yourself looking like Cher if you're a five-foot-tall blonde such as myself. There's also no sense in seeing yourself as Brooke Shields if you are three times her age. The idea is to picture the best possible *you*, not the best possible someone else.

You can imagine yourself looking younger and slightly taller, however, because as you shape up, posture and skin tone improve, along with energy levels. But keep your expectations realistic.

One of the best ways to get a realistic idea of how you want to look is to take a front and back photograph of yourself—close enough to get a clear view of your entire body. The next step is to "fix" the picture. Draw over each body part and correct it into the form you wish to achieve.

Next, stand in front of the mirror in the nude or in your underwear, and picture your body metamorphosing and evolving into that corrected picture. Take time to analyze each of your nine body parts as you stand in front of the mirror.

Start at the top of your body and work your way down. First look at your shoulders. Imagine them becoming well shaped rather than stooped and hunched. Now look at your chest. See muscles forming under your breasts, making your breasts fuller and higher. Imagine the new cleavage that will soon become evident.

Next, look at your arms. See them beginning to take on a shapely look. Imagine your biceps developing to give your arm a curvaceous feminine muscle. Hold out your arm and wave it back and forth. Picture the flabby triceps hardening into a solid muscle that will never wobble again.

Look at your stomach. See the little pot melting away and being replaced by small, sensuous muscles. Look at the front of your thighs. See the cellulite smoothing out and being replaced by a shapely quadriceps muscle.

Now use a hand-held mirror to observe your back. Look at your shoulder and upper back muscles. Imagine your rounded back forming sexy lines of definition. Look at your lats. See a shapely "V" taking the place of your straight, shapeless back, and your waist looking smaller as a result.

Now look at your buttocks. Imagine them being lifted and tightened. See round, firm buttocks replacing soft flabby ones. Observe the back of your thighs. See the sagging cellulite disappearing. Finally, look at your calves. Imagine a curvaceous, shapely muscle forming under your skin, making your leg look perfectly balanced.

Does this sound like a lot of magical thinking? Well, it isn't. It would be if you then just sat around all day and ate potato chips and watched TV. But since you're going to be working out—hard—and following a low-fat eating plan, of course it will happen. It will happen in time. But in order to speed up the event, and to give yourself courage, visualize in the mirror.

When you stop to think of it, you already have proof that such things happen. Who among us has not had the experience of running into an old friend we haven't seen in over a year who lost so much weight that he or she looked like a different person. Think of visualization as a sped-up process of what really happens. That's all it is—seeing the result ahead of time.

How often should you visualize this way? At least once a week. You will need to do this in order to encourage yourself. You should also do it whenever you catch yourself looking in the mirror and putting yourself down. Instead of allowing your mind to continue on a track such as, "Look at that fat stomach,

28 you pig," immediately begin to visualize the fat melting away and shapely, sexy muscles forming.

DECIDE HOW LONG IT WILL TAKE YOU TO GET IN SHAPE

Before you start your workout and eating plan, it's a good idea to decide how long it will take you to get in shape. First, read chapter 2 and read the generalized expectations. Then adjust those general expectations to your particular energy and personality. Here's how.

Look in the mirror and ask yourself, "How long do you need to get into shape?" An answer will come to you. Your subconscious mind knows the answer. Be calm and listen to your inner voice.

You may come up with "three months," even though the plan says you can do it in six weeks. Your inner voice may be telling you that you need the extra time—that you don't want to rush yourself. If that's the case, go with the flow of your subconscious. It's better to follow your natural pace than to feel obligated to fit into a standard regimen.

On the other hand, your inner voice may indicate to you that you have the energy and motivation to do it in four weeks, even though the plan says six weeks. If this is so, follow that lead. Your subconscious knows what you are ready for and how much energy you will be willing and able to invest.

Next, set the date. Count from the day you are going to begin the workout, and mark your in-shape date on the calendar. Then look in the mirror and tell your body to get in shape by that date. When you go to bed, just before you fall asleep, think about that date and rest in the knowledge that on that date your body will be transformed into its goal shape.

Your subconscious mind will assist you in getting to your goal. The subconscious works somewhat like a homing torpedo. It will help you to zig-zag your way around obstacles to get to your goal. For example, there will be days when you have made up your mind not to work out, even though you know you should. Suddenly, for seemingly no reason, you jump up and get going. Why is this? It's your subconscious mind remembering that it has a job to do—to get you to your goal by a given date, no matter what. Bodybuilders have known this truth for a long time. In fact, we count on it to get us into shape by a certain day for big events—photo shoots, television appearances, and contests. It never fails. We've got it down to a science. I've given you the secret here.

VISUALIZE AS YOU EXERCISE

To further add to your progress, focus your attention on the muscle you are exercising, rather than just letting your mind wander as you work out. Look directly at the muscle you are exercising. Touch it if you can. Picture the excess surrounding fat melting away, and imagine a tight, toned, shapely muscle forming.

The more mental cooperation you give your body, the more quickly it will get into shape. You can speed your progress as much as 50 percent if you use your mind to cooperate.

YOUR MIND CAN TELL YOUR BODY WHAT TO DO

There's even more that you can do. You can actually order your body to get in shape. As you are exercising, "tell" your body certain things. Tell the fat to go away. Tell the muscles to take shape and to form in perfect symmetry. Instruct your body to meet the specifications you have outlined as you envisioned yourself in the mirror.

VISUALIZE YOURSELF BEING IN CONTROL OF WHAT YOU EAT

Teach yourself to stop overindulging in fattening foods. Picture yourself eating your favorite fattening food until you can hardly get up out of your chair. Imagine yourself feeling nauseous as you walk away from the table.

Now get another picture of yourself. See yourself confronted with the same food. This time, picture yourself eating a medium-size portion of the food. Then imagine yourself about to have a second helping. See yourself suddenly experiencing a flashback—a flashback of the way you felt the time you overindulged. Then picture yourself pushing away the second helping and getting up from the table with a knowing smile and a feeling of triumph.

This method works surprisingly well for those who try it. The problem is, so many people think it sounds foolish, so they dismiss the idea without giving it a fair trial. I have never met one person who tried this method and said it did not help. It always helps, but you have to put in the preconditioning time. It will only take a few minutes, and you can do it any time of the day or night. You can do it while you're lying in your bed at night, when you're riding in a car, or even when walking in the street. You don't have to close your eyes to do it. You can picture the foods in your mind.

People have cured themselves from overeating, overdrinking, and overdoing many things. Visualization is used successfully even in life and death situations such as helping patients to combat cancer.

You can use the same method to help you to begin enjoying nutritious foods, foods that previously held no interest for you. Imagine a table full of fresh, steamed vegetables, broiled fish or chicken, and colorful fruits.

See yourself sitting down to the table with a voracious appetite. Imagine yourself selecting from these fine foods and eating until you are satisfied. Now see yourself rising from the table with vitality and joy. Picture yourself feeling strong and energetic.

The next time you are in the supermarket, or in a restaurant, you may surprise yourself by choosing healthful foods you had never considered eating before. It will be visualization, or mental preconditioning, at work.

MAKE A SIMPLE SIX-WEEK COMMITMENT

Make the commitment to yourself. Promise yourself that, come what may, you will pick a start date and stick to this program for six weeks, no matter what happens. Make this a non-negotiable issue. Promise yourself that even if nothing seems to be happening, you will work for six weeks. Promise yourself that no matter what thoughts go through your mind, you will still work out according to the schedule you have picked.

AN ADDED BONUS: IMPROVED SELF-ESTEEM

If you make this commitment and keep it, you will gain more than just an in-shape body. Your self-esteem will improve. You will feel empowered as you see that by taking specific action you were able to change the shape and feel of your body. This knowledge will help you to realize that you can also effect changes in other areas of your life. Instead of feeling helpless in personal or career-related situations, you will find yourself believing that you can effect changes there, too.

WORKING OUT BEATS DEPRESSION

If you are angry or frustrated and pick up the weights and start working out, you quickly realize that you have a wonderful outlet for your frustration. With each repetition, you let go of some of the built-up tension as you vent your spleen on the workout. In fact, many people deliberately hit the weights with the very purpose of relieving accumulated tension.

But to pick up the dumbbells and start working out when you are not angry or frustrated but just plain down in the dumps, depressed, is another matter altogether. Those are the times when you have the blues to such an extent that you simply don't have the energy even to be angry. You experience a helpless sense of lethargy, to the point where you don't have the will even to move. Your world appears gray and bleak. Your thoughts are negative. You just don't care about anything. What should you do at times like these?

I have a challenge for you. I want you to wait until you are in the worst possible mood—one like I've just described, or worse. Then, in spite of anything you feel or think, by a sheer act of will, pick up the dumbbells and begin to do your workout. You will feel horrible. You won't want to do it. But do it just as an experiment. Instruct your arms and legs to move, to go through the motions as if in a robot-like state.

If you do this, what will happen? After working out for about five minutes, your mood will subtly change. Somehow you will feel strangely different. You won't know at exactly what moment it happened, because you will be in constant motion, caught up in the intensity of the workout. By the time you are finished, whether it be twenty, thirty, or forty minutes later (depending upon which workout you have chosen), strangely enough, you will no longer be depressed. In fact, you will be rather mellow, almost happy. Then suddenly you will remember how awful you felt before, and you'll think, "Isn't it amazing?"

But what's really amazing is that it happens every time. You can bet on it. There's a scientific reason for this mood change. It has been discovered that exercise helps the body to release chemicals called endorphins into its system, which affect specific areas of the brain and spinal cord in a positive way. In fact, when analyzed under laboratory conditions, it was discovered that these chemicals have an effect on the body and mind very similar to that of an opiate. In other words, exercising in a vigorous manner, as described in this workout, gives you a natural high. It helps you to look at the world through sunnier glasses, so to speak. Perhaps it is for this reason that psychologists have been recommending exercise to their depressed patients for years.

Once you experiment and find out for yourself that it is true, you may think your problems are over. Whenever you're depressed you'll remember how great you felt the last time you exercised and easily be able to overcome any temptation not to work out. *Wrong*. When you're feeling depressed, the sensation is so overpowering that you will still be very tempted to lie there in lethargy and let the mood have its way. However, having experienced the wonderful mood-changing effect of exercise, you will at least know that it does work, and this recollection will help you to perform what will still be an act of will— moving from point A to point B to pick up the dumbbells and start working out.

IF ALL ELSE FAILS, *JUST DO IT!*

There will be times when no motivation works. You just don't want to work out, and that's that. Well, my final word on this subject is, when all else fails, *just do it*. Remember, thoughts are just that, only thoughts. Temptations. If you don't give in to them, no harm has been done. *It's what you do that counts*, not what you almost didn't do. So no matter what thoughts you are battling, as long as you work out anyway, it doesn't matter if you were bombarded with all sorts of negative thoughts. Once you start moving those dumbbells, the victory is yours.

STICKING POINTS ARE WHEN YOU'RE MAKING THE MOST PROGRESS

There may come a time during your workout when nothing seems to be happening. But a lot is happening. You really are making progress, only the results are not visible yet. Just as you don't know exactly the point at which a child grows, you don't always know when your body is losing fat and gaining muscle. You work out and you stick to your diet, but it seems nothing is happening. Then one day you look in the mirror and you see a difference. You try on a pair of pants that were previously too tight in the hip-buttocks area, and now they fit. Why? When did this happen?

Slowly. When nobody was watching. Perhaps when you were sleeping—the way nature usually works. So don't expect to see results every day. There may be a few weeks at a time when you see nothing. But hang in there. It's happening. Believe me.

LIGHTEN UP

You've been beating yourself half to death for having committed the heinous crime of enjoying a few pitiful doughnuts, a chocolate bar, or a greasy hamburger, all of which you're convinced went straight to your hips. It's a dismal self-accusation—you are very bad to seek a little pleasure in food.

But when you think of it, aren't you being a little hard on yourself?

In his book *Healthy Pleasures*, Dr. Robert Ornstein writes, "When confronted with a threatening situation, animals have essentially two choices: to flee or to fight. Humans have a third alternative: to laugh."

Let's learn to laugh at ourselves. Let's not forget to keep things in perspective. All we are trying to do is win the battle of the bulge, not World War III. By learning to step back and laugh at yourself, you make it easier to succeed. You relax. You realize that unless your doctor has told you otherwise, it's not a life-or-death issue. It's something you want to do for yourself. And with a little luck and a lot of determination, you will do it.

Surprisingly, once you step back and get things into perspective, mysteriously, instead of complaining, you become motivated. Why? Your strength is no longer being sapped by guilt and self-condemnation. Your energy is released for action—and you take action.

LET'S NOT BE FANATICS

I am not a "health nut." I never have been and I never will be. I drink coffee (two to three cups a day), I occasionally drink champagne and vodka or other alcohol, and I indulge in bagels and cream cheese and other fat-promoting foods from time to time.

If I couldn't enjoy my life, being in great shape would be a shameful waste. I want to have fun; I don't want to spend all my waking hours thinking about diet or training. After all, the purpose of getting in shape is to be able to stop obsessing about being fat and go on with our lives. With the Fat-Burning Workout, you don't have to be in a panic that at any moment all your progress will suddenly evaporate.

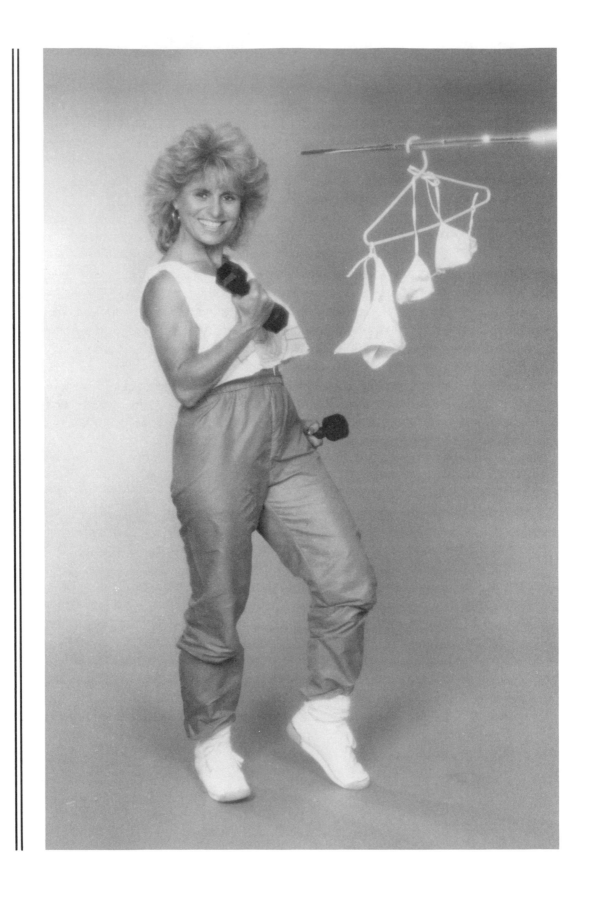

4 | DEFINITIONS

This is a chapter on details. It presents the basic exercise terms used in connection with this workout. Chances are you're already familiar with some of the material contained in this chapter. For example, if you've read any of my workout books or worked out with weights before, you already know the meaning of words like *set* and *repetition.* You may even know what it means to *pyramid* the weights and to use the *split routine.*

If you do, all well and good. You may skim over those parts of the chapter. But do not completely skip them, because I've used specific examples from the Fat-Burning Workout in illustrating the definitions. In other words, reading through the definitions will serve as a preview of the workout.

You should also not neglect to review the section describing muscles and their action. After reading about the muscles of each of the nine body parts involved in this workout, locate them first on the anatomy photograph, then on your own body. This will help you to visualize the evolution of your body into its desired form.

EXERCISE

There are seven exercise expressions you will need to know in order to follow this workout. They are: *exercise, repetition, set, rest, routine, workout,* and *resistance.*

An **exercise** is a given movement for a specific muscle, designed to cause that muscle to grow and become stronger. For example, the dumbbell bench press is an exercise designed to shape and strengthen the chest, or pectoral, muscles.

A **repetition,** or "rep," is one complete movement of an exercise, from start, to midpoint, to finish. (The finish position is actually back to start.) For example, one repetition of the dumbbell bench press involves raising the dumbbells held at either side of the chest area (in start position) until your arms are extended straight up with the dumbbells held above the chest area (midpoint), then moving back to start. (See page 81 for photographs illustrating this exercise.)

A **set** is a specified number of repetitions of an exercise performed without a rest. In this workout, you will be performing twelve repetitions for your first set of each exercise, ten repetitions for your second set of each exercise, and eight repetitions for your third set of each exercise.

A **rest** is a pause between sets or exercises. The purpose of the rest is to allow the working muscle enough time to recuperate so that it can efficiently perform the work of the next set. When working with heavy weights, a rest period of thirty to sixty seconds between sets is usual. Since this is a special fat-burning program, using light weights, very little rest time is allowed.

A **routine** is the specific combination of exercises prescribed for a given body part. For example, the regular Fat-Burning Workout chest routine includes the incline dumbbell press, the incline dumbbell flye with a twist, and the cross-bench pullover.

A **workout** includes all of the exercises to be performed on a given day. For example, on the first day of the Fat-Burning Workout, you exercise your upper body: biceps, chest, shoulders, triceps, and back. On the second day, you exercise your lower body: thighs, buttocks, abdominals, and calves.

The term *workout* can also be used to describe the overall exercise program.

Resistance refers to the heaviness of the weight used in a given exercise. Since this is first and foremost a fat-burning workout and not a bulk-building workout, you will be using lighter weights—less resistance—than you would use in a regular body-building workout. For example, for your first set of twelve repetitions of the dumbbell press, you will use three pounds of resistance, where a bodybuilder might use fifteen. Less resistance allows you to work faster and so burn more fat, at the expense of building larger muscles.

TECHNIQUE

There are twelve expressions of technique you need to know to follow this workout. They are: *aerobic, anaerobic, intensity, muscle isolation, split routine, contract, flex, stretch, regular pyramid, modified pyramid, progression*, and *burn*. There are three other expressions of technique which are crucial to this workout: the *giant set*, the *super-giant set*, and the *monster set*. To avoid repetition, I have saved the description of these expressions for the next chapter, where I tell you how to perform the Fat-Burning Workout.

An **aerobic** exercise is a physical fitness activity that can be sustained by your body's own, natural supply of oxygen and that causes your pulse to reach a rate of between 70 percent and 85 percent of its capacity and stay there for twenty minutes or longer. Some medical experts now feel that even a sustained heart rate of 60 percent achieves an aerobic effect. If you perform this workout as prescribed, you will be well within the aerobic range.

Anaerobic activity is too demanding to be supported by the body's natural oxygen supply, and so creates an oxygen debt. When this happens, the exerciser is forced to take a rest literally in order to "catch her breath." Power lifting is an example of an anaerobic activity.

Although regular weight training has traditionally been considered to be an anaerobic activity, if done as prescribed in this workout, it becomes an aerobic activity. How can this be? The continual, steady flow of movement using light weights allows the body to maintain enough oxygen to sustain the activity. In this sense, this workout can be compared to circuit training (see page 7).

Intensity is the degree of difficulty of the exercise program you are following. Intensity can be increased by increasing the number of repetitions, increasing the load of weight, or reducing the rest periods allowed between sets and between exercises. The Fat-Burning Workout is a high-intensity program because you are allowed only a few short rest intervals.

Muscle isolation is the method of exercising a body part independently of other body parts. In order to ensure maximum growth and development, shaping and strengthening a given body part, it is necessary to provide that body part with uninterrupted work. In other words, it is not okay to do one exercise for the biceps and then skip to a shoulder exercise, and so on. All the exercises for one body part must be completed before the exercises for another body part are begun. In this workout, you are required to perform a minimum of three exercises for a body part before moving to the next body part.

The **split routine** is the technique of working only certain body parts on a given day. A routine can be split into two or three workout days. The split routine allows muscles the required seventy-two hours' rest before they are challenged again. If not allowed time to recuperate, muscles may become exhausted from overtraining, and development may be hindered. In fact, you might actually wear away developing muscle by overtraining.

In this workout, the routine is split into upper and lower body workouts. The upper body—biceps, chest, shoulders, triceps, and back—is exercised on workout day one. The lower body—thighs, buttocks, abdominals, and calves—is exercised on workout day two.

When you **contract** a given muscle, you shorten the muscle fibers of that muscle by squeezing them together. For example, you contract your chest muscles when performing the dumbbell bench press as you raise your arms up to the fully extended position. In that position, you can feel your chest muscles condense, or "crunch," together.

When you **flex** a muscle, you take contraction a step further. You give the contracting muscle an extra, willful "squeeze." Using the above example, when your arms are in the up position, and your chest muscles are contracted, instead of just returning to the down position, you pause for a split second and deliberately squeeze your chest muscles as hard as you can.

When you **stretch** a given muscle, you lengthen the muscle fibers. For example, when performing the dumbbell bench press, you stretch your chest (pectoral) muscles when you return from the arms-straight-up position (the contracted or flexed position) to the start position.

The **pyramid system** of weight training involves the addition of weight and the reduction of repetitions with each set until a peak is achieved, then the reduction of weight and the addition of repetitions until the final set is identical to the initial one. The system is more readily understood with a simple example.

Set 1: twelve repetitions at three pounds
Set 2: ten repetitions at five pounds
Set 3: twelve repetitions at three pounds

The **modified pyramid system** of weight training involves the addition of weight and the reduction of repetitions for each set until the peak of the pyramid is reached. The set ends there. The continual progression of weight allows the muscle to be challenged to work up to capacity, ensuring optimal development. In this workout we will be using the modified pyramid system. Here is a typical example.

Set 1: twelve repetitions at three pounds
Set 2: ten repetitions at five pounds
Set 3: eight repetitions at ten pounds

Progression refers to the occasional adding of weight to specific exercises when the weights being used for those exercises are no longer enough of a challenge. For example, in this workout you will be using light weights overall in order to cope with the intensity of the workout. However, after a while (perhaps in a month) these weights may feel *too* light. When this happens, it's time to add weight to your overall routine. For example, instead of using three pounds for your first set of repetitions for your biceps routine, you may decide to use five pounds. For your second set, you may find that ten pounds is best, and for your third set, you may find that you can now handle fifteen pounds. Your biceps routine may now look like this:

Set 1: twelve repetitions at five pounds
Set 2: ten repetitions at ten pounds
Set 3: eight repetitions at fifteen pounds

The expression **burn** refers to the feeling that you will sometimes get in your working muscle as the lactic acid builds up in the muscle tissue. This happens when the blood does not have enough time to carry the acid away as you work.

You may experience a burning sensation in your working muscle from time to time. Don't worry about it. It's a sign that you are working your muscle to the maximum. As your muscles get used to the workout, you will experience less and less of the "burning" sensation—unless, of course, you intensify your workout either by speeding it up or adding more weight.

PHYSICAL APPEARANCE

There are seven relevant terms relating to physical appearance. They are: *muscle mass*, *muscle growth*, *muscularity*, *definition*, *density*, *ripped*, and *symmetry*.

Muscle mass is the actual size of a given muscle. **Muscle growth** (hypertrophy) takes place over a period of time when the muscle is forced to lift progressively heavier weights. In order to grow extremely large, a muscle must be required to lift extremely heavy weights over a period of time.

Muscularity refers to the quantity of muscle in relation to fat. A sumo wrestler who weighs 400 pounds may have large, hulking muscles but low muscularity because large amounts of fat surround his muscles. On the other hand, a bodybuilder has high muscularity because a minimum of fat surrounds his or her muscles.

Definition means muscles are clearly delineated and visible. A muscle can only be well-defined when its lines are not obscured by the presence of fat. Those who follow this workout will have both a high degree of muscularity and, because of the reduction of fat, definition.

A muscle is said to have **density** when it is hard, as opposed to soft, and is packed with quality muscle fibers. The Fat-Burning Workout produces muscular density so that the body is firm and appealing to the touch, as opposed to soft and spongy.

A **ripped** muscle is one in which you can see superficial, slender lines separating the muscle from other muscles. For example, if a person has ripped deltoid (shoulder) muscles, one can see lines across that area. The "ripped" condition is an extreme of definition. Professional bodybuilders seek ripped muscles in order to win contests. Your muscles will be well defined but not "ripped."

Symmetry is the esthetic balance and proportion of muscles in relationship to other muscles on the body. It is the goal of this workout to provide the exerciser with near perfect symmetry. (There is no such thing as perfect symmetry on the human body. Our limbs are not exactly the same length, our feet are not the exact same size, etc.) Because near perfect symmetry is the goal, you should never exercise only selected body parts. You don't want to end up with well-developed arms and "chicken" legs, or muscular legs and "toothpick" arms. How sad it is to see a woman who is otherwise perfectly proportioned but has severely underdeveloped deltoid (shoulder) muscles. It gives her a stooped appearance and causes her to look years older.

EQUIPMENT

There are eight exercise equipment pieces that we will be referring to: the *flat bench*, the *incline bench*, *free weights*, the *dumbbell*, the *barbell*, the *plate*, the *collar*, and the *machine*.

The **flat exercise bench** is a standard padded bench that is parallel to the floor.

The **incline exercise bench** can be raised to an incline as high as a 45-degree angle. Since you will need both flat and incline exercise benches for this workout, it's a good idea to purchase a flat bench that can be raised to an incline. You may order such a bench from me. (see page 205.)*

Free weights are hand-held weights that can be carried about. Free weights include dumbbells, barbells, and exercise plates.

A **dumbbell** is a short bar (usually made of metal) that can be held in one hand and has raised, usually rounded ends. Most dumbbells have a permanently fixed weight on either end. I do not recommend dumbbells with removable plates. It takes too long to take them apart for readjustment, and the plates often loosen while you are using them.*

A **barbell** is a metal bar that is held in both hands, and that holds various weights on either end. Barbells come in weights from fifteen to forty-five pounds. You won't need a barbell or plates for this workout unless you choose to do the alternative exercises.

Plates are disc-shaped weights that can be placed on either end of a barbell or, in some cases, a dumbbell. They come in sizes as light as one and a quarter pounds, and go as high as forty-five pounds. If you choose to use the alternative barbell exercises presented later in the book, I suggest you purchase a fifteen-to-twenty-pound barbell and a set of two-and-a-half-pound plates, a set of five-pound plates, and a set of ten-pound plates. You probably won't need more than that.

A **collar** is a device placed on either end of the barbell or dumbbell to keep plates from sliding off. Placing and removing collars is time-consuming, and since I work with light weights, I never use them. Most bodybuilders don't. However, I advise you to use them, just to be on the safe side.

The exercise **machine** is a device designed to challenge one or more specific body parts. Years ago, Nautilus and Universal were virtually the only brands of machine available. Today, there are hundreds of brand names, including Cybex, Marcy, and Paramount.

Note: a flat exercise bench that raises to an incline, and three sets of dumbbells are all the equipment you will need for this workout.

WHY FREE WEIGHTS ARE SUPERIOR TO MACHINES FOR THE PURPOSE OF THIS WORKOUT

There is a distinct general advantage in using free weights as opposed to using machines, as well as specific advantages for the purpose of this workout.

To begin with, you can achieve greater flexibility by using free weights than you can by using machines. Most machines are not made to accommodate the smaller person, especially the smaller woman. They are built with the average-size man in mind.

Second, you can tighten and tone muscles more efficiently with free weights, since you are in complete control of the velocity and resistance of your movements. A machine does not allow for a full natural movement, no matter how efficient the machine. When you work with a machine, you lose a little bit of the workout, because the machine does some of the work. In my opinion, that's exactly why so many people love them.

Third, it is possible to burn a greater amount of fat by using free weights to exercise specific body parts because a free weight can be applied most directly to a specific muscle.

Fourth, whether working at home or in the gym, free weights are more convenient. They can be carried to one corner of the room and used there without disturbing other people.

Finally, free weights are more versatile. For example, you can work all nine body parts by using just one set of dumbbells. In order to work all nine body parts using machines, you would need enough machines to provide at least twenty-seven different exercises, since you must do at least three exercises per body part to get a complete workout. Most exercise machines provide only two or three exercises, so you'd need at least nine machines!

ADVANTAGES OF MACHINES OVER FREE WEIGHTS

Machines are usually considered safer than free weights because they are controlled by slides or cams and held in place by retaining pins. However, with the very light weights you will use with this workout, there is very little danger of self-injury.

Machines are also said to be time-savers because, in order to change their weights, all you have to do is move a pin up or down a notch. With free weights, you have to add plates to a barbell or pick up another set of dumbbells. Since this workout requires only three sets of dumbbells, it is at least as simple to use the dumbbells as it is to use the machines.

Machines are also said to be more efficient in isolating a muscle group for heavy overload. The Fat-Burning Workout does not seek to overload a muscle group, but to isolate a particular muscle and to work it to the maximum through an intense workout using light weights and short rest periods.

Much of the appeal of machines is their promise of "helping" the exerciser, and that's just what they do—help you. In my opinion, there are only a few exercise machines that are extremely valuable in helping to perfect the body shape. They are the lat pull-down machine, the pulley row, and the leg-extension/leg-curl machines. (If you belong to a gym, you might want to check them out.) However, there are free-weight substitutes for even these machines.

INJURY AND SORENESS

Muscle soreness is the result of microscopic tears in the fibers of the ligaments and tendons connecting the muscles, with slight internal swelling accompanying those tears. Such tears are perfectly normal. They are, in fact, necessary if you're going to make any progress in shaping and toning your muscles. If you didn't get any tears (or soreness) you wouldn't make any progress at all.

You can expect some soreness for the first few weeks. You'll learn to enjoy it as a signal that you're making progress. In fact, the soreness will excite you as you think about your developing body. Incidentally, the only way to make that soreness go away is to continue working out according to your schedule—soreness or no. If you stop working out, you will be back to square one when you start working out again, and you will have to go through it all again. The only thing to do is work through the soreness. If you work your sore muscles, they actually feel better than they do if you let them lie dormant and stiffen up further. The workout serves as a massage to your sore muscles. After working out for a few weeks, you'll probably experience little or no soreness.

Injury is easy to detect. Instead of the gradual soreness that comes as a result of normal working out, a sharp, incapacitating pain is experienced immediately. It is likely to stop you from working out even if you are foolish enough to try to continue. The most common injuries in weight training are tears to the covering of the muscle (the fascia), stretching and tearing of ligaments, and painful inflammation of a tendon (tendonitis).

If you are careful not to jerk or pull the weight in an abrupt manner, you will not only avoid fascia injuries but also avoid stretching or tearing of ligaments as well. In short, follow the exercise instructions carefully and you will have no problem. Although you are not allowed significant rests between sets, you are not required to rush through your repetitions. You should perform each rep carefully and deliberately.

Tendonitis is usually the result of lifting extremely heavy weights. If you break in gently and use the weights suggested in chapter 5, you are in no danger of incurring tendonitis. Power lifters and competitive bodybuilders are the ones most commonly afflicted with this ailment.

If at any time you think you are injured, *see your doctor immediately*.

MUSCLES

For your convenience, the following muscle descriptions are given in the order that you will find them in the exercise chapters. For example, on your first exercise day, you will work your biceps, chest, shoulders, triceps, and back, in that order. On your second exercise day, you will work your thighs, buttocks, abdominals, and calves. As you read the following descriptions, refer to the anatomy photographs on pages 45–46.

The **biceps** is the muscle that works to flex or bend the arm. It originates from the shoulder blade and terminates at the elbow. The "bump" that forms when you flex like Popeye is the biceps.

The **pectoralis major**, also referred to as the pectorals or "pecs," are the chest muscles used in all upper arm movement.

Don't confuse the pectoral muscles with the breasts themselves. The breasts are located on top of the pectoral muscle and are composed of fatty tissue. No amount of exercise can enlarge the breasts themselves. However, through proper exercise, the underlying pectoral muscle can be developed so that the breast is uplifted. In addition, appropriate pectoral work helps to develop the coveted look of "cleavage."

44

The pectoral muscles are fan-shaped. They spread out from the collarbone and run along the breastbone to the cartilage connecting the upper seven ribs to the breastbone.

The pectoral muscles are divided into a smaller "upper" (clavicular) and a larger "lower" (sternal) section.

The **deltoid** (shoulder) muscle works to raise the arm to shoulder height once the motion has been initiated by other muscles. It also assists in rotating, flexing, and extending the arm.

The deltoid muscle attaches in the upper area of the shoulder blade, where it joins the collarbone, and on the bone of the upper arm.

The **triceps** muscle works to extend the arm and the forearm. It attaches in three places, at the shoulder blade, the back side of the upper arm, and the elbow.

The **latissimus dorsi** are the large muscles that lend the back its "V" shape—its width. Well-developed "lats" help a woman's waist to appear small and minimize larger hips.

The latissimus dorsi work to pull the shoulders back and downward and the arm toward the body. The muscle on either side originates from the center of the back along the spinal column and extends to the tailbone. The muscle flares out into the shoulder area.

The **trapezius** muscle works to shrug the shoulder, to pull the head and shoulders back, and to support the shoulder blade when the arm is raised in an above-the-head position. "Traps" are usually highly developed in wrestlers and judo experts, as they are continually shrugging their shoulders in an effort to protect the neck against attack.

The muscle itself is triangular and flat. It originates along the spine and runs from the back of the neck to the middle of the back. The upper fibers of the trapezius are attached to the collarbone. For this reason, most people think of "traps" as being located between the neck and shoulder area, when in reality they are much larger than that. It is the visible part, however, that is located between the neck and collarbone. (See the anatomy photograph on page 46.)

The muscles of the hips and buttocks area are the gluteus maximus, gluteus medius, and gluteus minimus.

The **gluteus maximus**, which gives the buttocks its shape, is properly named, for it is usually the largest muscle in the body. It functions to rotate and extend the thigh. It is located behind the hip joint.

The **gluteus medius** is located just beneath the gluteus maximus. It functions to raise the leg out to the side and to balance the hips as weight is transferred from one foot to the other.

The **gluteus minimus** originates on the hipbone, and performs the same function as the gluteus medius.

The **quadriceps** (front thigh) muscle does the work of extending your leg from the bent position. It is composed of four muscles: the rectus femoris and

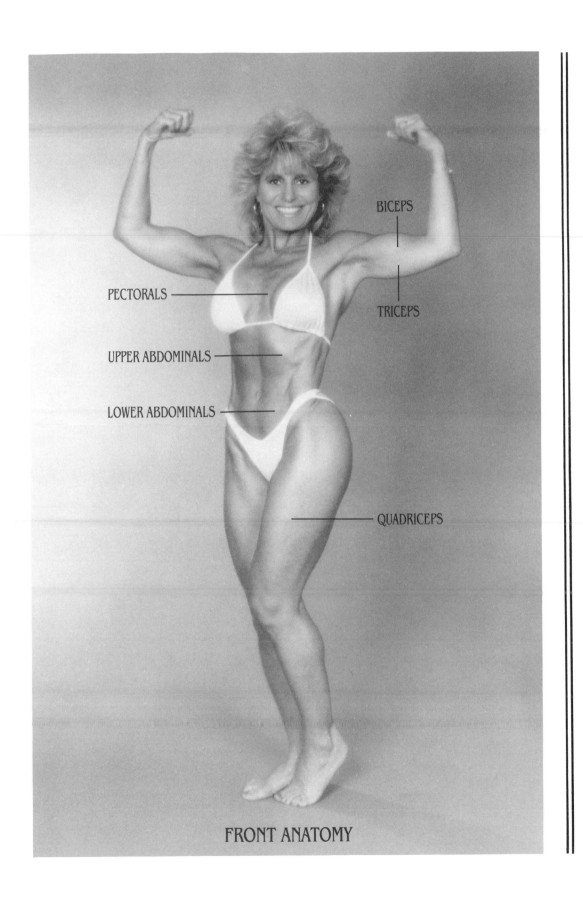

BICEPS

PECTORALS

TRICEPS

UPPER ABDOMINALS

LOWER ABDOMINALS

QUADRICEPS

FRONT ANATOMY

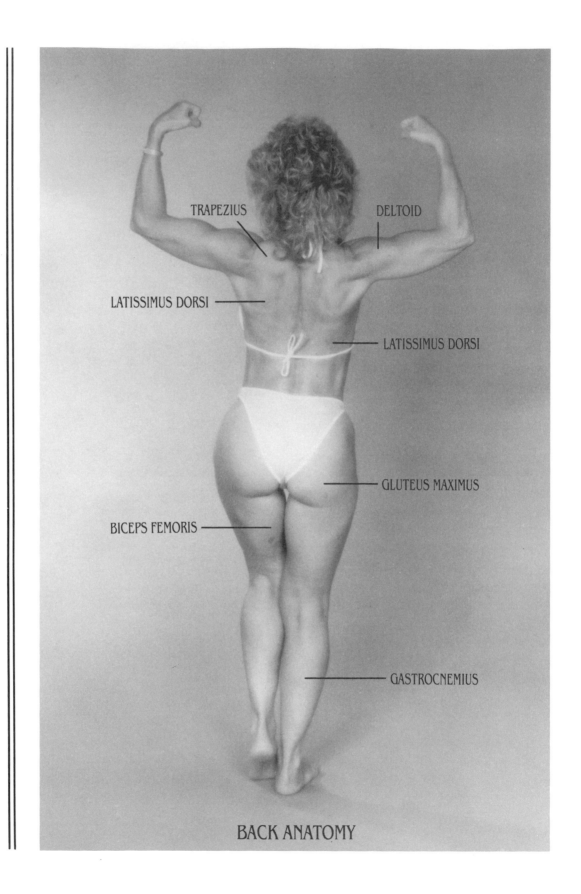

TRAPEZIUS

DELTOID

LATISSIMUS DORSI

LATISSIMUS DORSI

GLUTEUS MAXIMUS

BICEPS FEMORIS

GASTROCNEMIUS

BACK ANATOMY

three vasti muscles. The rectus femoris originates on a ridge on the front of the hipbone, while the three vasti muscles originate in various parts of the thigh bone. All four muscles come together at the kneecap.

The **hamstrings** (back thigh) muscles help to extend the hips, rotate the leg, and flex the knee. This is actually a muscle group composed of three muscles originating from the bony area of the pelvis. One, the biceps femoris, is a two-headed muscle on the outer thigh. The other two, the semimembranosus and the semitendinosus, are connected at the inner knee.

The primary stomach muscles, or **abdominals**, are really a single muscle, the rectus abdominis, a long, powerful, segmented muscle that works to pull the torso or upper body toward the lower body when sitting up from a lying down position. The "abs" originate from the fifth, sixth, and seventh ribs and run up and down the abdominal wall. Although the rectus abdominis is technically one long muscle, we usually refer to its "upper" and "lower" sections for purposes of exercise.

The last two muscles exercised in the Fat-Burning Workout are those in the calf of your leg—the gastrocnemius and the soleus.

The **gastrocnemius** helps to bend the knee and flex the foot downward. It connects in the middle of the lower leg and ties in with the Achilles tendon. The point where its two segments are connected or tied together forms what we see as the calf muscle.

The **soleus** functions to flex the foot downward, but it does not help to bend the knee, since it doesn't cross the knee joint. It is located directly beneath the gastrocnemius muscle.

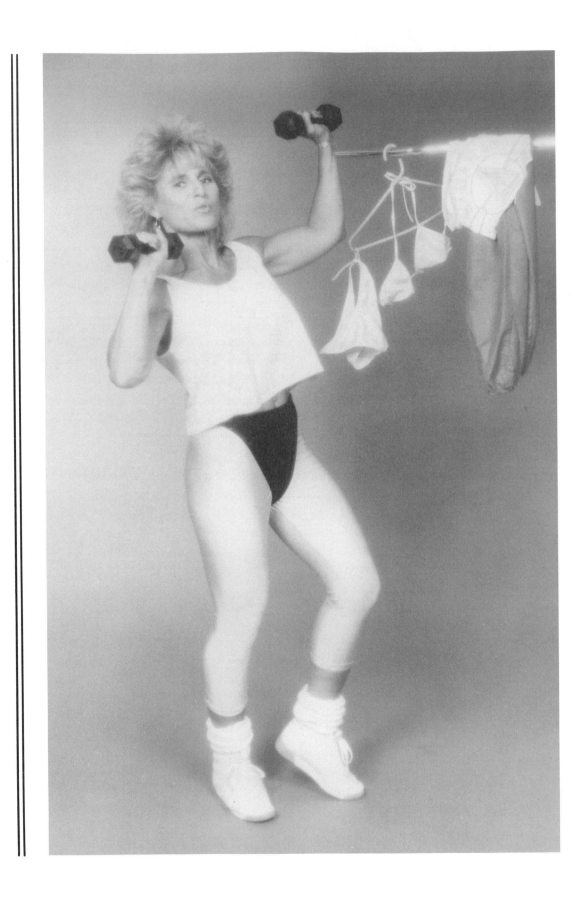

5 | HOW TO DO THE FAT-BURNING WORKOUT

The Fat-Burning Workout is exciting. You work through it quickly and you're out of there. It can be done at home or in a gym. It's a no-nonsense workout, designed only for those who mean business. In this chapter, you'll learn the difference between the three choices you have: the regular Fat-Burning Workout, the Intensity Fat-Burning Workout, and the Insanity Fat-Burning Workout. Your choice will depend upon how much time you have to invest, but no matter which workout you choose, you will get results in record time. (See chapters 6 and 7 for directions on performing all exercises mentioned in this chapter.)

THE REGULAR FAT-BURNING WORKOUT— 20 MINUTES

This workout is based upon the *giant set*. If you've used a regular body-building program, you know that the usual method of working out is to perform three or four exercises per body part, and to do about three sets for each of those exercises. In such a routine, you do all three sets for one exercise before advancing to the next exercise, and you rest about thirty seconds between each set.

When using the giant set, however, you perform your first set of all three exercises for a given body part without resting. Only then do you rest—but only for ten to fifteen seconds before going on to the second set of all three exercises. Here's how the method works for your biceps muscle.

Biceps Routine

1. Standing alternate dumbbell curl
2. Standing angled simultaneous dumbbell curl
3. Standing alternate hammer curl

You do your first set of standing alternate dumbbell curls then, without resting, do your first set of standing angled simultaneous curls. Without resting, you move on to your first set of standing alternate hammer curls. Only then do you rest, but not for long—only for ten to fifteen seconds.

Then, following the modified pyramid system, you pick up a slightly heavier weight and do your second set—with fewer repetitions—again working through all three exercises before taking a short ten-to-fifteen-second rest. Finally, you do your last set of all three exercises without resting, using a slightly higher weight and doing a few less repetitions.

Let's spell it out exactly:

Biceps Routine

1. Standing alternate dumbbell curl
2. Standing angled simultaneous dumbbell curl
3. Standing alternate hammer curl

Set 1: *Twelve repetitions* for each of the three exercises—no rests between sets. Use three-pound dumbbells.

Rest ten to fifteen seconds.

Set 2: *Ten repetitions* for each of the three exercises—no rest between sets. Use five-pound dumbbells.

Rest ten to fifteen seconds.

Set 3: *Eight repetitions* for each of the three exercises—no rest between sets. Use ten-pound dumbbells.

Rest ten to fifteen seconds.

After you complete your first body part routine, you move to the next routine for that day. In this case, it is the chest routine.

Chest Routine

1. Incline dumbbell press
2. Incline dumbbell flye with a twist
3. Cross-bench pullover

You will proceed exactly as described above. Do the first set of twelve repetitions for each exercise, using the three-pound dumbbells, then rest for ten to fifteen seconds. Then do your second set of ten repetitions for each of the exercises, using the five-pound dumbbells. After you've finished your second "giant set," rest again for ten to fifteen seconds. Then you do your final giant set of eight repetitions for each exercise, using the ten-pound dumbbells. Rest for ten to fifteen seconds, and then move on to the next body part—shoulders.

By now you know the basic system. It's the giant set: three separate exercises without resting. You'll use this method throughout the Fat-Burning Workout.

Here is a list of all the exercises you will be doing if you choose the regular Fat-Burning Workout—the easiest and least time-consuming of the three workout choices. (See chapters 6 and 7 for directions for performing each exercise. See pages 62–63 for weight selection.)

Regular Fat-Burning Workout—Day One
Upper Body Workout:
Biceps, Chest, Shoulders, Back, Triceps

(giant sets—three exercises per body part)

Biceps

1. Standing alternate dumbbell curl
2. Standing angled simultaneous dumbbell curl
3. Standing alternate hammer curl

Chest

1. Incline dumbbell press
2. Incline dumbbell flye with a twist
3. Cross-bench pullover

Shoulders

1. Standing side lateral
2. Standing front lateral
3. Pee-wee lateral

Triceps

1. One-arm overhead triceps extension
2. One-arm triceps kickback
3. Flat cross-face triceps extension

Back

1. Reverse bent dumbbell row
2. Bent dumbbell shrug
3. Dumbbell upright row

Regular Fat-Burning Workout—Day Two
Lower Body Workout:
Thighs, Buttocks, Abdominals, Calves

Thighs

1. Regular squat
2. Lunge
3. Sissy squat

Buttocks

1. One-legged butt lift
2. Lying butt lift
3. Feather kick-up

Abdominals

1. Sit-up
2. Leg raise
3. Lying leg-in

Calves

1. Seated straight-toe calf raise
2. Seated angled-out-toe calf raise
3. Seated angled-in-toe calf raise

THE INTENSITY FAT-BURNING WORKOUT— 30 MINUTES

The Intensity Fat-Burning Workout is exactly the same as the regular Fat-Burning Workout, except, as you might have guessed, you must do more work. Instead of doing giant sets, you will be doing *super-giant sets*. A super-giant set is just a bigger giant set. It consists of four exercises instead of three. Everything else remains exactly the same. The work is harder because you have to do four sets instead of three before resting. For example, in your biceps routine, you now have this added exercise—the concentration curl. Your biceps routine now looks like this:

Biceps Routine

1. Standing alternate dumbbell curl
2. Standing angled simultaneous dumbbell curl
3. Standing hammer curl
4. Concentration curl

The method is the same: perform the first set of each exercise with no rest before proceeding to your second set, and so on.

Once you become familiar with the exercises, you will see how convenient it is to go from one exercise to the next. You don't even have to move off your spot. You stand in one place with the dumbbells. The only difference in each exercise, except for the last one, is the way you move the dumbbells. And even for the last one, the concentration curl, all you do is bend over. How convenient!

Here is a complete list of your Intensity Fat-Burning Workout exercises:

Intensity Fat-Burning Workout—Day One
Upper Body Workout:
Biceps, Chest, Shoulders, Back, Triceps

(super-giant sets—four exercises per body part)

Biceps

1. Standing alternate dumbbell curl
2. Standing angled simultaneous dumbbell curl
3. Standing alternate hammer curl
4. Concentration curl

Chest

1. Incline dumbbell press
2. Incline dumbbell flye with a twist
3. Cross-bench pullover
4. Flat dumbbell flye

Shoulders

1. Standing side lateral
2. Standing front lateral
3. Pee-wee lateral
4. Bent lateral

Triceps

1. One-arm overhead triceps extension
2. One-arm triceps kickback
3. Flat cross-face triceps extension
4. Incline cross-face triceps extension

Back

1. Reverse bent dumbbell row
2. Bent dumbbell shrug
3. Dumbbell upright row
4. Seated dumbbell back lateral

Intensity Fat-Burning Workout—Day Two
Lower Body Workout:
Thighs, Buttocks, Abdominals, Calves

Thighs

1. Regular squat
2. Lunge
3. Sissy squat
4. Front squat

Abdominals

1. Sit-up
2. Leg raise
3. Lying leg-in
4. Crunch

Buttocks

1. One-legged butt lift
2. Lying butt lift
3. Feather kick-up
4. Prone butt lift

Calves

1. Seated straight-toe calf raise
2. Seated angled-out-toe calf raise
3. Seated angled-in-toe calf raise
4. Standing straight-toe calf raise

THE INSANITY FAT-BURNING WORKOUT— 40 MINUTES

The Insanity Fat-Burning Workout is exactly the same as the above workouts, only you will be doing even *more work*. Instead of doing giant sets or super-giant sets, you will now be doing *monster sets*. Instead of doing three or four exercises per body part, you will be doing five exercises per body part (except for three body parts that do not benefit from such intensive training).

You follow the same pattern as described above, doing all five first sets before resting and proceeding to all five exercises for your second set, and so on. The six body parts for which you will do monster sets are: chest, shoulders, back, thighs, buttocks, and abdominals. If you did five sets for the smaller biceps, triceps, and calf muscles, you would be in danger of overtraining them, and you might wear away, rather than build up, firm muscle tissue.

So if you choose to perform the Insanity Fat-Burning Workout, you will be doing only six, rather than nine, additional exercises in total. The routine may not actually take a full ten minutes extra. Perhaps this will motivate you to be daring enough to try it.

Since your first Day One exercise series, biceps, requires only four exercises, nothing will change here, so let's use the second Day One exercise series, chest, for an example.

Chest

1. Incline dumbbell press
2. Incline dumbbell flye with a twist
3. Cross-bench pullover
4. Flat dumbbell flye
5. Flat dumbbell press

Exactly as described in the preceding pages, you will do your first set of each exercise consecutively with no rest. You will not be allowed to take advantage of your pitiful ten-to-fifteen-second rest until you have performed all five sets (the first set of each exercise done in succession).

Here is a complete list of your Insanity Fat-Burning Workout exercises:

Insanity Fat-Burning Workout—Day One
Upper Body Workout:
Biceps, Chest, Shoulders, Back, Triceps

(monster sets—five exercises per body part)

Biceps

1. Standing alternate dumbbell curl
2. Standing angled simultaneous dumbbell curl
3. Standing alternate hammer curl
4. Concentration curl

Chest

1. Incline dumbbell press
2. Incline dumbbell flye with a twist
3. Cross-bench pullover
4. Flat dumbbell flye
5. Flat dumbbell press

Shoulders

1. Standing side lateral
2. Standing front lateral
3. Pee-wee lateral
4. Bent lateral
5. Standing alternate dumbbell press

Triceps

1. One-arm overhead triceps extension
2. One-arm triceps kickback
3. Flat cross-face triceps extension
4. Incline cross-face triceps extension

Back

1. Reverse bent dumbbell row
2. Bent dumbbell shrug
3. Dumbbell upright row
4. Seated dumbbell back lateral
5. Lying dumbbell back lateral

Insanity Fat-Burning Workout—Day Two
Lower Body Workout:
Thighs, Buttocks, Abdominals, Calves

Thighs

1. Regular squat
2. Lunge
3. Sissy squat
4. Front squat
5. Leg curl

Abdominals

1. Sit-up
2. Leg raise
3. Lying leg-in
4. Crunch
5. Standing serratus crunch

Buttocks

1. One-legged butt lift
2. Lying butt lift
3. Feather kick-up
4. Prone butt lift
5. Scissors

Calves

1. Seated straight-toe calf raise
2. Seated angled-out-toe calf raise
3. Seated angled-in-toe calf raise
4. Standing straight-toe calf raise

PLAN "B"—SPEED SETS FOR CONVENIENCE OR EMERGENCY

In a speed set, you perform all three sets of a given exercise the way you would in a regular body-building workout, pyramiding the weights as usual. But—and herein lies the difference—you do not take any rest between sets. You take your ten-to-fifteen-second break only after you have completed the entire exercise of three sets.

What is the purpose of a speed set? It can be used when it is impossible to do giant sets, super-giant sets, or monster sets. At times you will find that you can do the first three of your exercises as a giant set, but for some reason, it is inconvenient to incorporate that fourth exercise into your giant set.

There are several instances in which the speed set is useful:

58

▪ Use the speed set when the position is awkward.

You may find that in certain cases, it is awkward to incorporate a given exercise into the super-giant or monster set. For example, you may have no trouble performing the first four exercises of a given routine using the super-giant set method, but when it comes to the fifth exercise, you may find that the positioning of that exercise causes you to waste too much time. The insanity thigh routine is an example.

1. Regular squat
2. Lunge
3. Sissy squat
4. Front squat
5. Leg curl

For the first four exercises, there is no problem moving quickly from one exercise to the other, because you are standing for each of them. However, when it comes to the last exercise, you must leap onto the floor, lie on your stomach, and place the dumbbell between your feet. This wastes a little time, and it may break your sense of momentum. So, for the thigh routine, you may want to do your first four exercises as a super-giant set and then speed-set the last exercise. You can alter your routine whenever you prefer to use a speed set. You will lose nothing in terms of the fat-burning effect.

▪ Use the speed set for your buttocks and abdominal areas.

Some women find that they like to speed-set the entire buttocks and abdominal routines, rather than perform them in giant sets, super-giant sets, or monster sets. They enjoy getting the full feel of each individual exercise before moving to the next exercise.

Try to exercise your buttocks and abdominals as described in the standard program, but feel free to experiment with speed-setting these two body parts.

▪ Use the speed set when equipment isn't available or cannot be monopolized.

The most important instance in which you may utilize the speed set is in the case where you are working out in a gym and some of the equipment necessary for your exercises is not available all at once. (This is more likely to happen if you choose to use the alternatives suggested for the gym workout, in which machines are involved.)

The wise thing to do here is speed-set as many exercises as are necessary, especially if the gym is crowded. It's better than standing guard over the equipment like a growling dog.

WEIGHTS USED IN THIS WORKOUT

In the beginning, I suggest that you use the following weights for all exercises:

Set 1: three-pound dumbbells
Set 2: five-pound dumbbells
Set 3: ten-pound dumbbells

Note: You may want to start with threes, fives and eights if you think you are not strong enough to handle the ten pounds.

You will probably have no trouble with these weights for biceps, chest, and back. However, you will most likely not be able to lift more than the three-pound dumbbells for your shoulders and triceps until you have been working out for at least a month, as these are weaker muscles. If this is the case, simply do not pyramid the weights until you are strong enough to do so. You may still do fewer repetitions for each set, as described in the pyramid system.

Some of you will feel that three-pound dumbbells are too light for the biceps, chest, and back right from the beginning. If so, you may adjust the weight to suit your present strength level. You may want to use ten-pound, twelve-pound, and fifteen-pound weights for biceps, chest, and back. However, I doubt that you will unless you have been weight training for years.

When to Raise Your Overall Weights

If you are using the weights suggested above—three, five, and ten pounds—after a few months, the weights may feel too light for you. You will know that they are too light when the weights seem to offer little or no resistance as you move them and you feel as if you didn't get a real workout when you're finished.

When you feel that your weights are too light, go up a few pounds all around. In other words, instead of using threes, fives, and tens, use fives, eights, and twelves for that exercise.

The Highest You Should Go

Even if you have been working out for years, doing a regular body-building routine, I don't recommend going any higher than twenty pounds for your

60

highest weight for any exercise in this routine. Why? If you go too heavy, you will slow yourself down. (You will find yourself wanting to take longer rests than are advised.) This is a fat-burning/muscle-shaping workout, not a bulking-up routine. There is no need to go really heavy—ever.

Buttocks and Abdominals Require Little or No Weight, but Higher Repetitions

Those of you who have worked with other body-building routines already know that as a rule, buttocks and abdominals are not exercised with any significant weight. These two areas are favorite places for fat accumulation. In order to stimulate maximum fat loss in these areas, it is necessary to use little or no weight and do many repetitions.

Eventually, you will be doing fifteen to twenty-five repetitions per set for each of the buttocks and abdominal exercises. In the beginning, however, chances are you will only be able to do three to five repetitions per set. Don't be discouraged. Even if you add only one repetition each time you work out, you will be doing a full set of fifteen in a matter of weeks.

If You Do Not Wish to Purchase More Than One Set of Dumbbells

You may be reluctant to purchase more than one set of dumbbells at this time, yet you want to begin working out. Instead of pyramiding the weights, you may use one set of three- or five-pound dumbbells for all sets of all exercises. Instead of doing twelve, ten, and eight repetitions per set, do ten repetitions for all sets.

This method may be a little boring, because you will never alter your repetitions or weights, but it does work to burn maximum fat, as long as you follow the method exactly in every other way. You will not build quite as much muscle, however, as you would if you followed the modified pyramid system, but you will see a major change in your body.

BREAKING IN

This is an extremely intense routine. You will have no trouble whatsoever doing it, however, if you carefully follow the advice given in the following paragraphs and break in *gently*. If you are foolish, however, and insist upon doing the entire workout the first week, you will become so sore you may be tempted to quit. So please, please, please—be patient. It will only take you three weeks to break in.

Breaking In If You Have Already Been Working Out

If you have recently been following a workout such as the one I describe in *Now or Never, Hard Bodies, Perfect Parts, The Hard Bodies Express Workout,* or *The Twelve-Minute Total-Body Workout,* you need not break in as gently as others, unless you choose to. All you really have to do is take longer rests for the first two weeks. Instead of taking no rests between sets, take fifteen-second rests between sets and thirty-second rests between body parts for the first week. For the second week, take ten-second rests between sets, and twenty-second rests between body parts. For the third week, you can follow the routine exactly. You may do this whether you choose the regular, the Intensity, or the Insanity routine.

You may choose whatever weight is comfortable for you. Chances are you will be able to use weights that are between one-third and half of what you used before. Feel it out. I would stick to the lighter weights in the beginning, just to get used to the routine and to avoid getting discouraged.

Breaking In If You Have Never Worked with Free Weights but Are in Good Aerobic Shape and Basically Strong

Consider the first few weeks a warmup. Follow this modified plan, concentrating on learning the basic movements of the exercises.

Week 1: first set of each exercise
Week 2: first and second set of each exercise
Week 3: all three sets of each exercise (the regular Fat-Burning Workout)
Week 4: advance to Intensity workout (optional)
Week 5: advance to Insanity workout (optional)

Do not strain yourself. Remember, if you find the five- and ten-pound weights too heavy, stick with the threes until you feel that the threes are too easy and you are ready for fives and, later, for tens. There is no rush here. If the threes are heavy for you, you are working just as hard as a person who uses fives and finds them heavy. Your effort is measured by how hard *you* are working, not by the actual weight you are lifting. (By the way, if even the threes are too heavy for you, you may get one- or two-pound dumbbells. Easy does it. In time you will be stronger than you could ever have imagined. Just take one step at a time.)

Breaking In If You Have Never Worked with Free Weights, Are Not in Aerobic Shape, and Are Very Weak

It will take you a little longer to break in. You should not work with weights for the first three weeks. Instead, do all the exercises by simply moving your body through the exercise movements. That will be enough of a challenge to your muscles initially. Then, after three weeks, introduce the weights. Here's how your break-in schedule will look.

Week 1: Set 1, no weights

Week 2: Sets 1 and 2, no weights

Week 3: Sets 1, 2, and 3, no weights

Week 4: Set 1 only, three pounds, twelve repetitions

Week 5: Sets 1 and 2 only

        Set 1: three pounds, twelve repetitions
        Set 2: three pounds, ten repetitions

Weeks 6—10: Sets 1, 2, and 3

Set 1: three pounds, twelve repetitions
Set 2: three pounds, ten repetitions
Set 3: three pounds, eight repetitions

Week 11: Begin to use the modified pyramid system (see page 38 for review). Do this only as you feel strong enough.

STRETCHING

There's good news. You don't have to stop and do a special group of stretches for this workout. Why? Because your first, lightest-weight set provides a natural stretch. If you wish, you may do three repetitions of each exercise for that workout day with no weight before beginning your workout. I don't find it necessary to do that. The choice is yours.

SHOULD YOU WORK OUT AT HOME OR IN A GYM?

The beauty of this workout is that you need so little equipment that you can work out at home without a problem. I enjoy going to the gym, but at times I get so busy I simply can't spare the travel and changing time. If I work out at home, I save myself at least an hour. Sometimes that means the difference between working out or not working out. On days like that, working out at home is a lifesaver.

If you do work out in a gym, at first you may worry about monopolizing too much equipment. If you look closely at the workout, however, you'll quickly realize that won't be a problem. All you really need for the entire workout is three sets of dumbbells (unless you choose to do some of the alternatives).

Just go to the dumbbell rack, claim your dumbbells by carrying them off into a corner, and begin to work. If anyone comes over and asks if you're using all the dumbbells, just say, "Yes, I'm giant-setting; I'll be finished in a few minutes." Then keep going. You will be using only one set at a time, but you will require the other dumbbells for final sets.

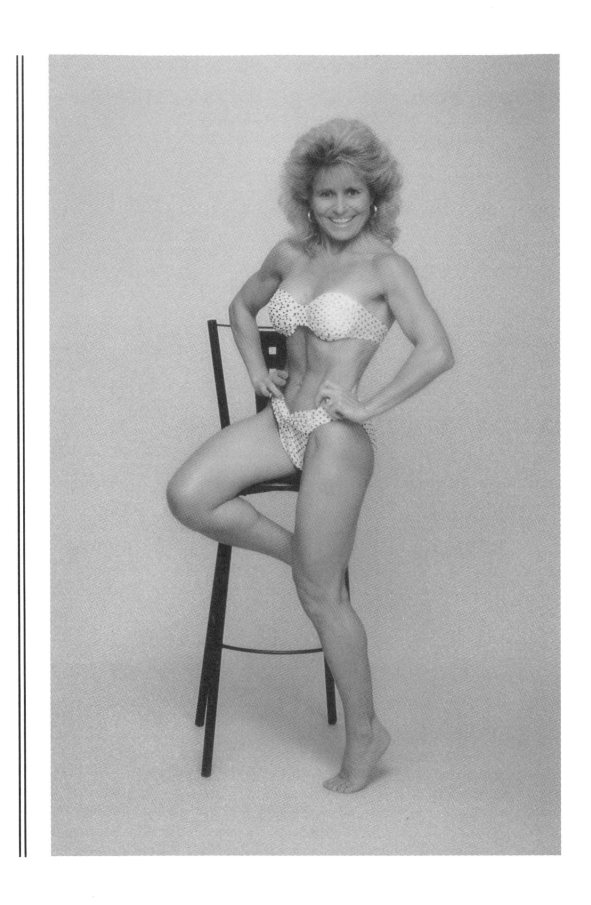

I've done this workout in gyms all across the United States. I've come into a gym as a stranger, scanned the situation, and secured my equipment. I've always been able to work out. In the worst situation, when a particular person was clearly annoyed that I was "hogging" the equipment, I made a deal: We "worked around" each other. People are reasonable If you show them respect. If there was a problem, I just went into Plan B, speed-setting my exercises instead of doing monster sets. So what? I still got my fat-burning effect.

This worked even when I used the gym alternatives, such as the barbell and the incline and regular bench press, and cable rows for the back. No matter what happens in a gym, once you have the necessary piece of equipment, you can always speed-set because then you are using it nonstop (except for a split second when you change your weights) and you have "squatter's rights." Who can say a word about that? In fact, most people will get out of your way because you'll give the impression that you are a real pro.

The Advantage of Working Out at Home

Of course, there is a distinct advantage to working out at home. No one can bother you. You're the boss. You can do your workout in peace without anyone threatening your equipment. You can play your own music. (I like to play "Hooked on Classics" and get wild.) Naturally, you will have to use self-control and let the answering machine pick up your calls, ignore the doorbell, and tell whoever else that is home, you are not available   and mean it.

Also, you save travel time. In some cities, it's more than that. In the winter, it can get so cold that you just don't feel like going out of the house again once you get home. The mere thought of venturing out into the vicious wind is enough to make you skip a workout. It's so wonderful to be able simply to walk into the next room and begin working out.

Finally, if you're going to work at home all the time, you save money on a gym membership.

The Advantage of Working Out in the Gym

For me, the main advantage of going to a gym is the camaraderie. I enjoy seeing the same old faces sweating it out day after day, just like me. It makes me see that I'm not alone, and that comforts me. It actually makes me feel secure to know that there are others who plod to the gym day after day, week after week, month after month.

66

There are days when I'll go to the gym and not even say a word to anyone. Just a nod or a glance or a quick grunt of acknowledgment is enough for me. But just the same, I feel great having been in the presence of other dedicated exercisers. In addition, as mentioned before, there are a few very useful machines in the gym that are too expensive for home purchase.

If You Choose to Work Out in the Gym— Taking Advantage of the Alternatives

If you choose to work out in the gym, take careful note of the alternatives listed at the bottom of each exercise. Many of these alternatives suggest the use of barbells or machines that are not available to you at home.

All Things Considered

I take whichever advantage suits me. I work at home and in the gym— whichever is convenient. When I go to the gym, I perform the alternative exercises, taking advantage of the gym equipment. But the fact is, for this workout you don't really need the gym. The choice is completely yours.

HOW MANY DAYS A WEEK SHOULD YOU WORK OUT?

The ideal number of days to work out is four or five a week. However, if you can't spare four days a week, you will see tremendous results even if you work out only three days—but it may take you a little longer to reach your goal.

If you are eager to get to your goal faster and have the time and energy, you can work out five or six days a week. This will speed up your progress.

SPACING YOUR WORKOUT DAYS

The ideal thing to do is to space your workout days as evenly as possible. For example, if you're only going to work out three days a week, it would be best if you could leave a day between workouts. However, with this workout, it isn't absolutely necessary to do that, because you are working on a "split routine," and enough rest time is allowed between body parts even if you work two days in a row.

If you are working out four days a week, the ideal thing to do would be to work every other day, and two days in a row one time. For example, you might work Monday, Wednesday, Friday, and Saturday. If you are working out five days a week, the ideal arrangement is never to leave more than one day without working out. Work in any combination except five days in a row.

These are the ideal situations. But who has the luxury of building her life around her workouts? I certainly don't. I work out four days a week, and I fit those four days in wherever I can. If I have to, I work four days in a row and don't work out for the other three days. I try not to let this happen all the time, but if it does, so be it. The beauty of this workout is that you have the flexibility of working out any time you want because of the split routine. This is a program made for busy women who have other responsibilities besides working out!

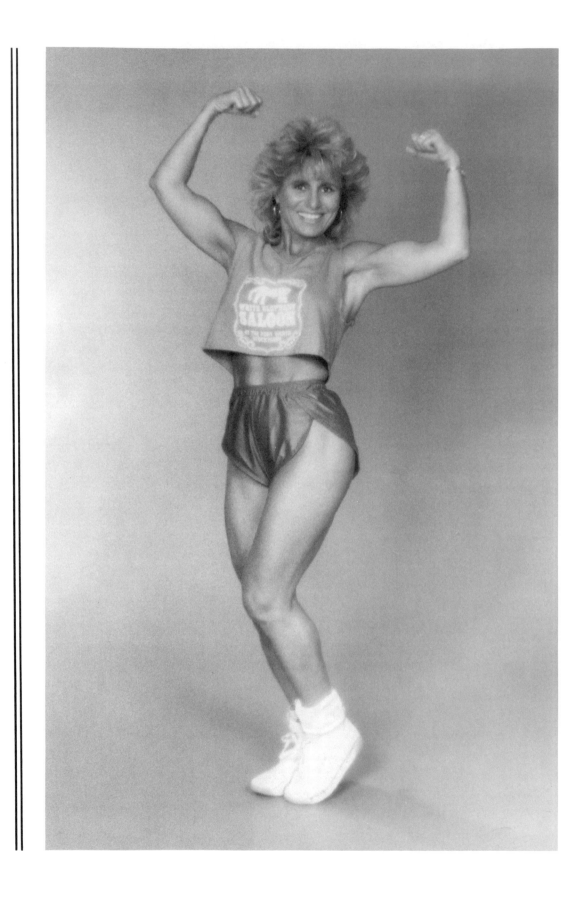

6 | THE UPPER BODY WORKOUT

This chapter contains the upper body workout. You will do this workout on alternate exercise days. If you choose to do the regular Fat-Burning Workout, do only the first three exercises for each body part, as described on pages 51–52. If you choose to do the Intensity Fat-Burning Workout, do only the first four exercises listed for each body part, as described on pages 53–54. If you are wild enough to choose to do the Insanity workout, do all exercises presented in this chapter.

WHY EXERCISE THE BODY PARTS IN THIS PARTICULAR ORDER?

The body parts exercised in this chapter are biceps, chest, shoulders, triceps, and back.

Biceps are easy to exercise. I've asked you to begin with something you can do without too much trouble. I also wanted to separate them from the other arm exercises, those for the triceps, so that you don't exhaust your arms.

The chest muscles are also an easy group to exercise, because the chest consists of large, strong muscles. In addition, a chest workout makes you feel strong and in control, and that will give you power for the rest of your workout.

Shoulders are traditionally exercised right after the chest because they are directly connected to the chest.

Your triceps, the other arm muscle, is exercised next because it is a relatively weak muscle, and I don't want you to save it for last. You may be too tired.

Your back is exercised last because the muscles there are not a difficult group to exercise. Also, after exercising your back, you are left with a feeling of total relaxation, which is a good way to end your workout for the day.

WHY DO THE EXERCISES FOR EACH BODY PART IN THE ORDER GIVEN?

There is also a method to my madness when it comes to the order of each particular exercise within the routine for each body part. The exercises are placed for body-positioning convenience. I make sure that, to the extent possible, I avoid asking you to do your first exercise standing, your second exercise on the floor, and your third exercise sitting. Where an exercise does require an awkward change in position, it is in the Intensity or Insanity workout (fourth and fifth exercises), so that it does not affect you if you're doing the regular Fat-Burning Workout. And, of course, if you are doing the Intensity or Insanity workout, you can always choose to isolate and speed-set the rare, oddly positioned exercise.

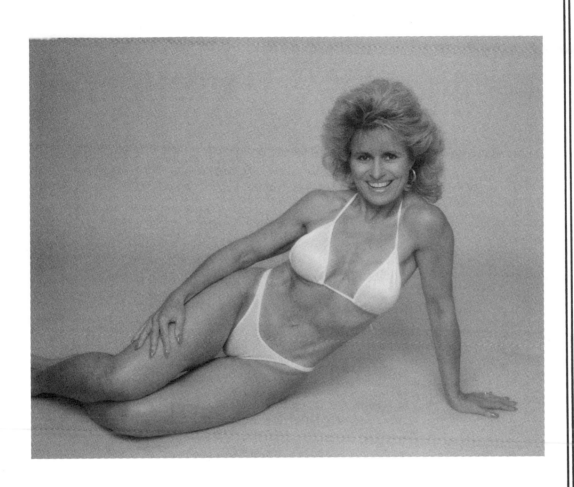

BICEPS ROUTINE

1. Standing Alternate Dumbbell Curl

This exercise develops and shapes the entire biceps muscle. In addition, it strengthens the forearm.

START: Stand with your feet together, holding a dumbbell in each hand, with your palms facing away from your body. Extend your arms at your sides.

ACTION: Keeping your arms close to your sides at all times, and your wrists locked and slightly bent upward, bend your left arm up until it reaches your left shoulder. As you begin to return to the start position, begin curling your right arm upward toward your right shoulder. Continue this alternate curling movement of the arms until you have completed your set. Without resting, begin the first set of your next biceps exercise, the standing angled simultaneous dumbbell curl.

ATTENTION: Work at an even and deliberate pace. Flex your biceps muscle on the upward movement, and let the muscle stretch out on the downward movement.

ALTERNATIVES: You may perform this exercise seated. You may perform this exercise on any double pulley machine.

STANDING ALTERNATE DUMBBELL CURL

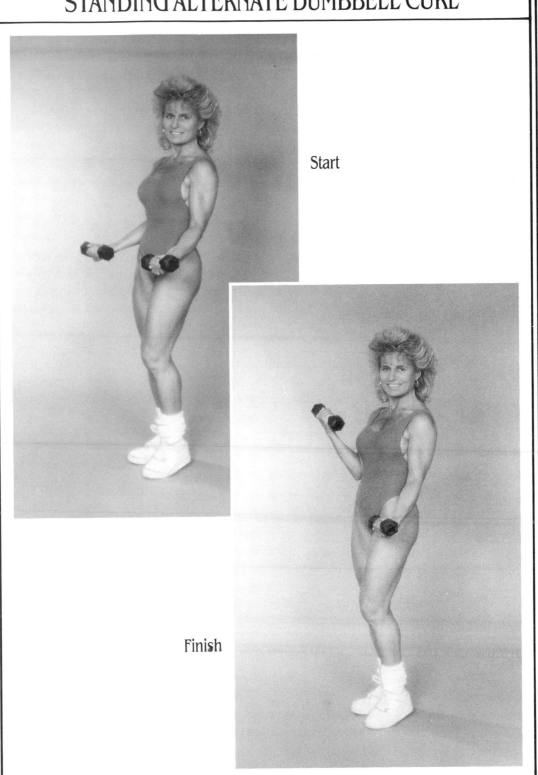

Start

Finish

2. Standing Angled Simultaneous Dumbbell Curl

This exercise shapes and develops the entire biceps muscle and strengthens the forearm.

START: Stand with your feet together with a dumbbell in each hand and palms facing away from your body. Place your arms at your sides and hold the dumbbells in a slightly angled out position.

ACTION: Keeping your arms close to your body, curl your arms upward simultaneously until you cannot curl them any further. Return to the start position and repeat the movement until you have completed your set. Without resting, begin the first set of your next biceps exercise, the standing alternate hammer curl.

ATTENTION: Do not rock your body back and forth as you curl and uncurl the dumbbells. Do not rush the exercise; rather, give each repetition the full range of movement. Half of a rep will work only half of a biceps.

ALTERNATIVES: You may perform this exercise with a barbell. You may perform this exercise on any biceps curl machine.

STANDING ANGLED SIMULTANEOUS DUMBBELL CURL

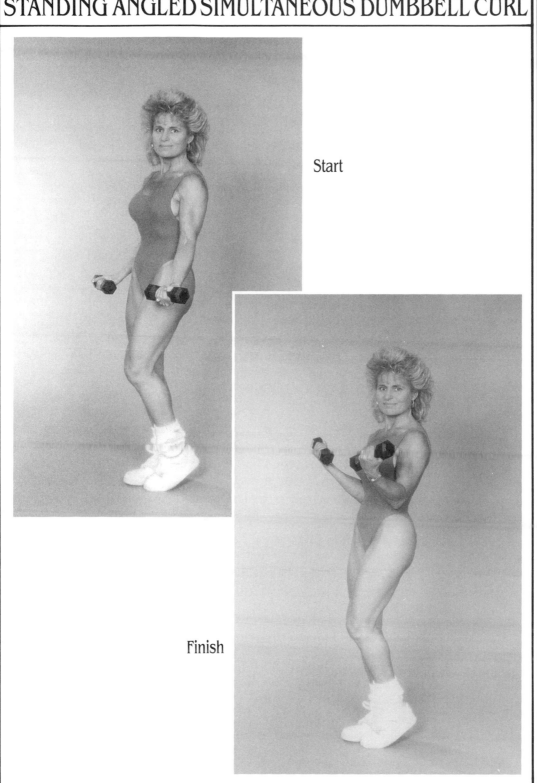

Start

Finish

3. Standing Alternate Hammer Curl

This exercise shapes and develops the entire biceps muscle. In addition, it strengthens the forearm.

START: With your feet together, hold a dumbbell in each hand, with palms facing your body, and let your arms hang down at either side of your body.

ACTION: With palms facing your body and the dumbbells in the "hammer" position (see photograph), curl your left arm up toward your left shoulder. As the dumbbell approaches your left shoulder, begin curling your right arm up toward your right shoulder; at the same time, uncurl your left arm. Continue this alternate curl movement until you have completed your set. If you are doing the regular Fat-Burning Workout, you may now rest for ten to fifteen seconds before beginning the second set of your first biceps exercise. If you are following either the Intensity or Insanity workout, without resting, begin your first set of the next biceps exercise, the concentration curl.

ATTENTION: Remember to flex your biceps muscles on the upward movement and stretch them on the downward movement. Don't rock back and forth with the movements. Keep your body steady. Don't rush this exercise. Remember, the idea is to limit rest periods, not to rush the repetitions.

ALTERNATIVES: You may perform this exercise seated. You may do simultaneous hammer curls.

STANDING ALTERNATE HAMMER CURL

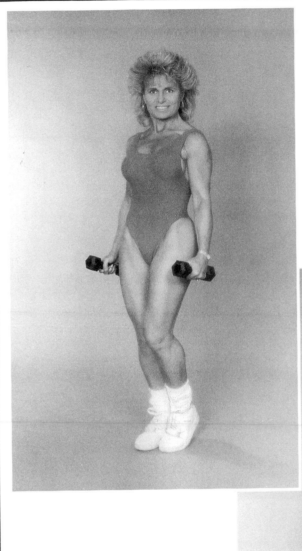

Start

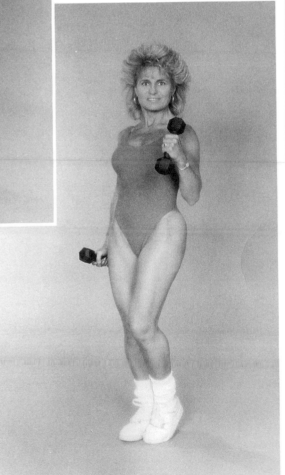

Finish

4. Concentration Curl

(for Intensity and Insanity workouts)

This exercise develops and shapes the peak of the biceps muscle. It also strengthens the forearm.

START: With your feet about two feet apart, bend over and position your right elbow on your right inner knee, holding a dumbbell with your palm facing away from your body and your arm extended straight down. You may support yourself with your right arm in any manner you choose. (This position grows on you. Trust me.)

ACTION: Curl your right arm upward until the dumbbell reaches approximate chin height. Return to the start position and repeat the movement until you have completed your set. Perform the set for your other arm. Rest ten to fifteen seconds and begin the second set of your first biceps exercise.

ATTENTION: Keep your elbow on your inner knee at all times. Flex your biceps muscle on the upward movement, and let it stretch out on the downward movement.

ALTERNATIVES: You may perform this exercise seated on a flat exercise bench.

CONCENTRATION CURL

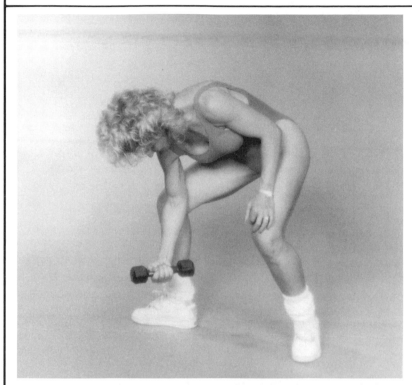

Start

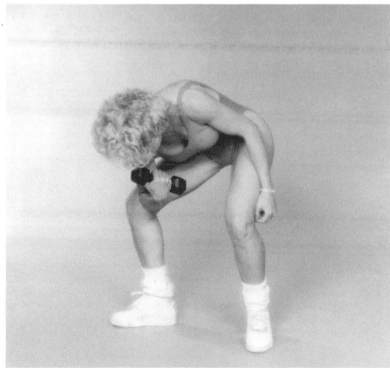

Finish

CHEST ROUTINE

1. Incline Dumbbell Press

This exercise develops and shapes the pectoral muscles, especially the upper chest area.

START: Lie on an incline bench with a dumbbell held in each hand and your palms facing upward. The outer edge of the dumbbells should be touching your upper chest area.

ACTION: Extend your arms upward until your elbows are nearly locked. The dumbbells should be in line with your upper chest in this fully extended position. Return to the start position and repeat the movement until you have completed your set. Without resting, begin to do the first set of your next exercise, the incline dumbbell flye with a twist.

ALERT: Maintain control of the dumbbells as you extend and lower your arms. Remember to flex your chest muscles on the upward movement and to stretch them on the downward movement. Don't hold your breath. Breathe naturally.

ALTERNATIVES: You may perform this exercise with a barbell.

INCLINE DUMBBELL PRESS

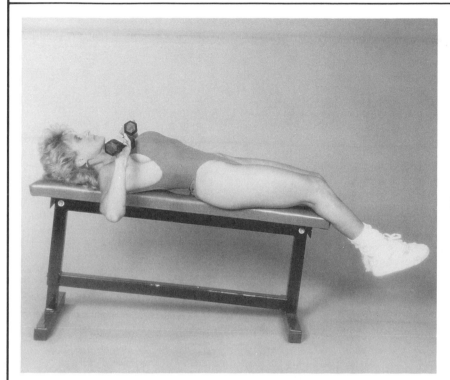

Start

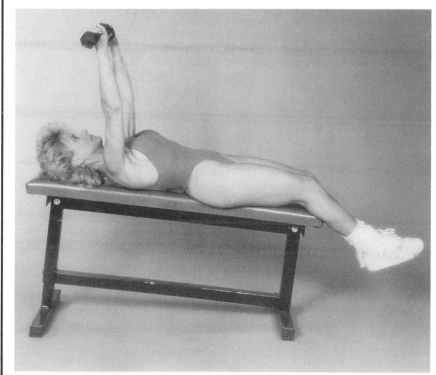

Finish

2. Incline Dumbbell Flye with a Twist

This exercise develops the chest (pectoral) muscles, especially the upper chest. It helps to create the look of cleavage.

START: With a dumbbell held in each hand and palms facing away from you, lie on an incline bench and extend your arms over your head so that the dumbbells are almost touching each other and are in line with the center of your chest.

ACTION: Extend your arms outward and downward in a semicircle until you feel a complete stretch in your pectoral muscles. As you return to the start position, turn your wrists inward, so that when you reach start position, the dumbbells are touching each other at the outer edge of their "bells." (See photograph.) Repeat the movement (remember to twist your wrists each time on the upward movement) until you have completed your set. Without resting, begin the first set of your next chest exercise, the cross-bench pullover. Remember to twist your wrists each time on the upward movement, because this is the movement that creates cleavage.

ATTENTION: Flex your chest muscles on the upward movement, and allow a full stretch on the downward movement. Be sure that your back remains firmly planted on the bench. Don't give in to the temptation to arch your back in an effort to make the work easier.

ALTERNATIVES: You may substitute any gym pec-deck machine for this exercise.

INCLINE DUMBBELL FLYE WITH A TWIST

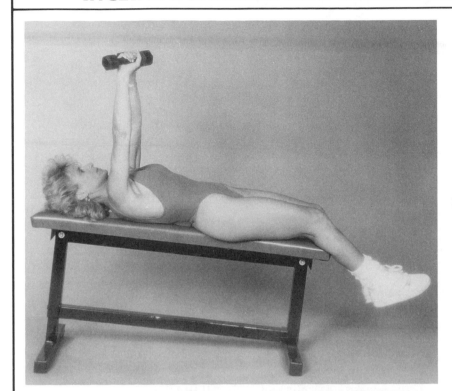

Start

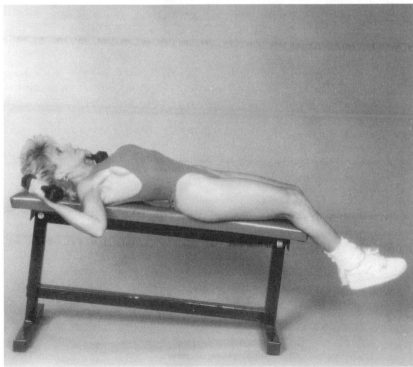

Finish

3. Cross-Bench Pullover

This exercise develops and shapes the entire chest area. In addition, it helps to expand the rib cage and stretch the shoulder muscles.

START: Place your shoulders at the edge of a flat exercise bench with your head extended over the bench. Place your feet flat on the floor and keep your buttocks as low to the ground as possible. Hold a dumbbell in your hands, palms upward, between your crossed thumbs. Extend your arms straight up so that the dumbbell is held directly over forehead.

ACTION: Lower the dumbbell behind you by lowering your arms and bending your elbows at the same time, until you cannot possibly go any farther. Feel a full stretch in your pectoral muscles and return to the start position. Flex your chest and repeat the movement until you have completed your set. If you are doing the regular Fat-Burning Workout, you may now rest for ten to fifteen seconds before beginning your second set of your first chest exercise. If not, proceed to your next exercise, the flat dumbbell flye, without resting.

ATTENTION: Remember to keep your buttocks as low to the ground as possible throughout the exercise. Do not rush. Work at an even pace. Keep your mind on your pectoral muscles as you work.

CROSS-BENCH PULLOVER

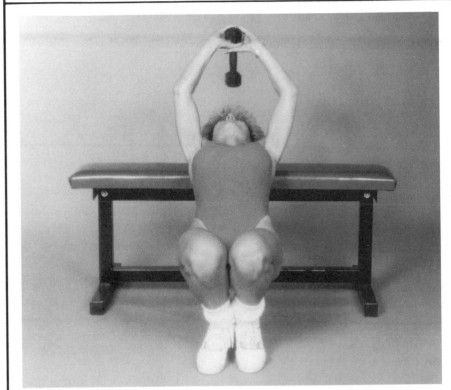

Start

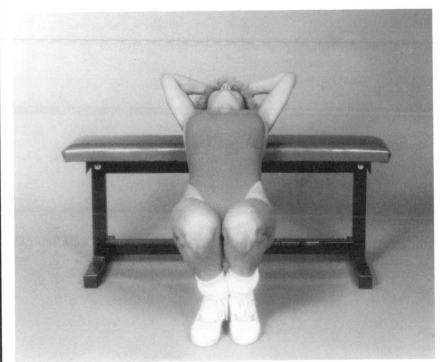

Finish

4. Flat Dumbbell Flye

(for Intensity and Insanity workouts)

This exercise develops and shapes the entire chest area.

START: Lie on a flat exercise bench with your arms fully extended and a dumbbell held in each hand and palms facing each other. The dumbbells should be touching each other, and in line with your chest.

ACTION: Extend your arms outward and downward in an arcing movement until you feel a full stretch in your pectoral muscles. Return to the start position, and flex your pectoral muscles. Repeat the movement until you have completed your set. If you are using the Intensity program, you may now rest for ten to fifteen seconds before beginning your second set of your chest exercises. If you are using the Insanity program, immediately begin the first set of your next chest exercise, the flat dumbbell press.

ATTENTION: Do not rush this exercise. Calmly extend and bring together your arms, stretching and flexing your pectoral muscles as you work. This can be a very relaxing exercise if you don't rush it.

5. Flat Dumbbell Press

(for the Insanity workout)

This exercise develops and shapes the entire pectoral area. Follow the instructions for the incline dumbbell press, only this time do the exercise on a flat exercise bench.

When you complete this exercise, you may rest for ten to fifteen seconds before beginning the second set of your first chest exercise, the incline dumbbell press.

FLAT DUMBBELL FLYE

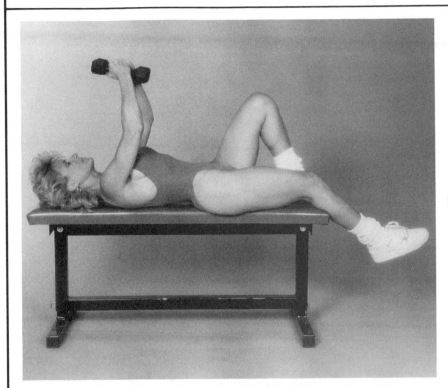

Start

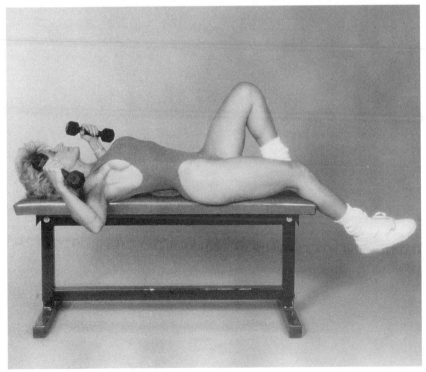

Finish

SHOULDER ROUTINE

1. Standing Side Lateral

This exercise develops and shapes the entire deltoid muscle, especially the side shoulder muscle.

START: Stand with your feet together. Hold a dumbbell in each hand, with your palms facing each other, and extend your arms downward, letting the dumbbells touch each other at the center of your body.

ACTION: Extend your arms upward and outward until the dumbbells reach slightly higher than shoulder height. Return to start position and repeat the movement until you have completed your set. Without resting, proceed to your next shoulder exercise, the standing front lateral.

ATTENTION: Beware of the temptation to swing the dumbbells out and up. Control your movements. Flex your deltoid muscles on the upward movement and allow them to stretch on the downward movement. Do not rush this exercise. Work deliberately and calmly.

ALTERNATIVES: You may perform this exercise while seated.

STANDING SIDE LATERAL

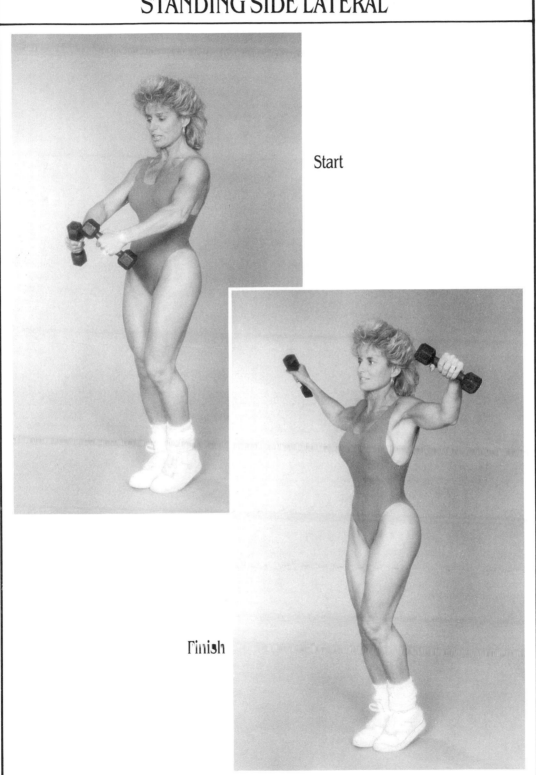

Start

Finish

2. Standing Front Lateral

This exercise develops and shapes the anterior (front) deltoid muscle.

START: Stand with your feet a natural width apart, holding a dumbbell in each hand, with your palms facing the front of your body. Extend your arms straight down so that the dumbbells are touching the center of your upper thighs.

ACTION: Lock your elbows and extend both arms upward until they are parallel to the floor. Feel the flex in your shoulder muscles, and return to the start position. Repeat the movement until you have completed your set. Without resting, proceed to the next shoulder exercise, the pee-wee lateral.

ATTENTION: Keep your arms close to the sides of your body at all times. Don't hold your breath. Breathe naturally.

ALTERNATIVES: You may perform this exercise by alternating arms. You may use a barbell instead of dumbbells.

STANDING FRONT LATERAL

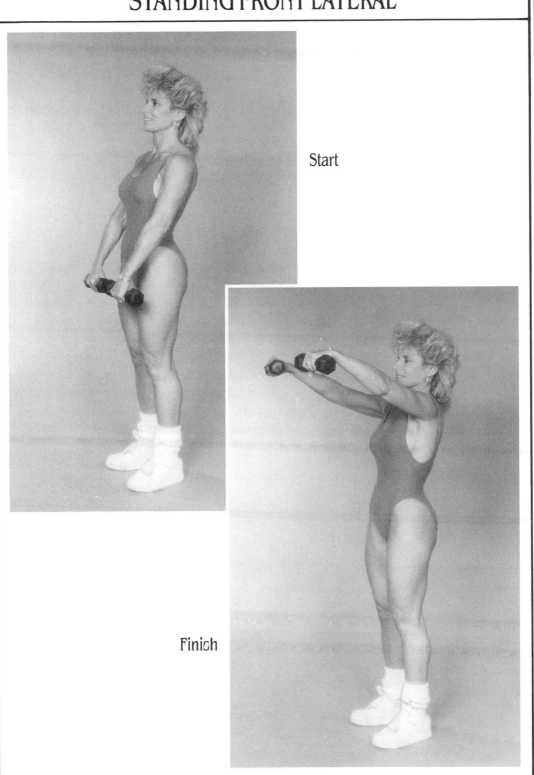

Start

Finish

3. Pee-Wee Lateral

This exercise develops and shapes the rear and side deltoid muscles.

START: Stand with your feet together, holding a dumbbell in each hand, with palms facing away from your body, and your arms behind your back. The ends of the dumbbells should be touching each other. Bend at the knees slightly and thrust your hips forward.

ACTION: Extend your arms outward and upward until the dumbbells reach ear-height and are at arm's length on either side. Return to the start position and repeat the movement until you have completed your set. If you are following the regular Fat-Burning Workout, you may take a ten- to fifteen-second rest before beginning the second set of your first shoulder exercise. Otherwise, without resting, begin the first set of your next shoulder exercise, the bent lateral.

ATTENTION: Remember to flex and stretch your rear deltoid muscles as you raise and lower the dumbbells. Do not rock your body back and forth as you work. Only your arms should be moving.

PEE-WEE LATERAL

Start

Finish

4. Bent Lateral

(for Intensity and Insanity workouts)

This exercise develops and shapes the rear and side deltoid muscle.

START: Stand with your feet together, holding a dumbbell in each hand, with palms facing each other. Bend over until your upper body is parallel to the floor and extend your arms straight down in front of you in the center of your body. Allow the dumbbells to touch each other at about knee height.

ACTION: Extend your arms outward until they are nearly parallel to the floor (your elbows can be very slightly bent in this position). Return to the start position and repeat the movement until you have completed your set. If you are using the Intensity routine, you may rest for ten to fifteen seconds before moving on to the second set of your first shoulder exercise. If you are using the Insanity routine, do not rest. Immediately begin your next shoulder exercise, the standing alternate dumbbell press.

ATTENTION: Keep your torso parallel to the ground throughout the movement.

ALTERNATIVES: You may perform this movement while lying facedown on a flat exercise bench.

BENT LATERAL

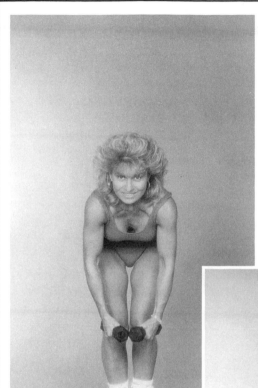

Start

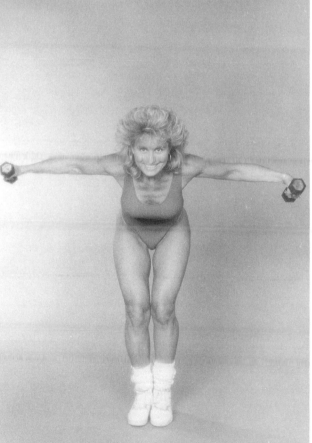

Finish

5. Standing Alternate Dumbbell Press

(for Insanity workout)

This exercise develops and shapes the entire deltoid muscle, with a special emphasis on the front deltoid muscle.

START: Stand with your feet together holding a dumbbell in each hand at shoulder height, with your palms facing away from your body.

ACTION: Raise your right arm upward until it is fully extended. While returning your right arm to the start position, begin raising your left arm upward until it is fully extended, while at the same time lowering your right arm. Continue this alternate up-and-down movement until you have completed your set. You may rest for ten to fifteen seconds before beginning the second set of your first shoulder exercise.

ATTENTION: Do not allow your torso to rock from side to side. Only your arms should be moving.

ALTERNATIVES: You may perform this exercise two arms at a time. You may perform this exercise on any gym shoulder-press machine.

STANDING ALTERNATE DUMBBELL PRESS

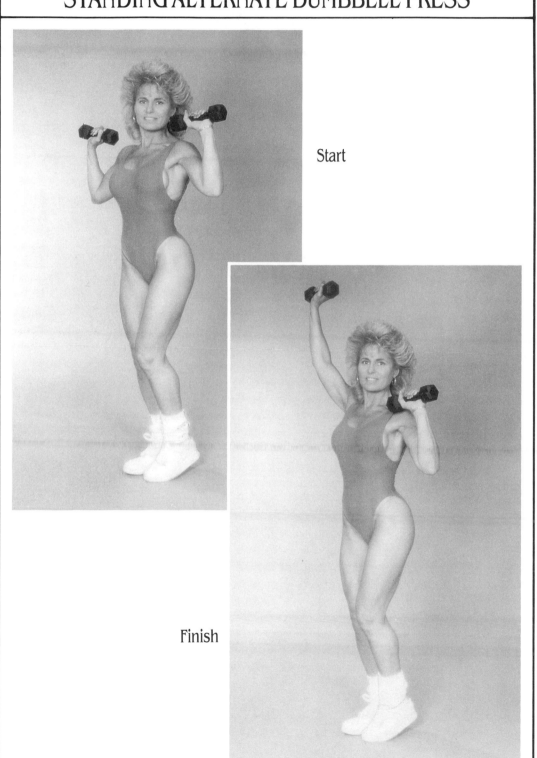

Start

Finish

TRICEPS ROUTINE

1. One-Arm Overhead Triceps Extension

This exercise develops and shapes the entire triceps muscle, especially the inner and medial heads of that muscle.

START: Stand with your feet together holding a dumbbell in your left hand, your palm facing your body and your arms extended straight up so that your upper arm is touching your ear.

ACTION: Lower the dumbbell behind your head until you cannot go any farther. Return to the start position and repeat the movement until you have completed your set. Repeat the set for your right arm then, without resting, move to your next triceps exercise, the one-arm triceps kickback.

ATTENTION: Keep your upper arm close to your head at all times. Be sure to bend your arm fully behind you on each downward movement, so that you feel a full stretch in your triceps muscle. Flex your triceps muscle on the upward movement.

ALTERNATIVES: You may perform this exercise using both arms with one dumbbell. (Naturally, you will use a heavier dumbbell in this case.)

ONE-ARM OVERHEAD TRICEPS EXTENSION

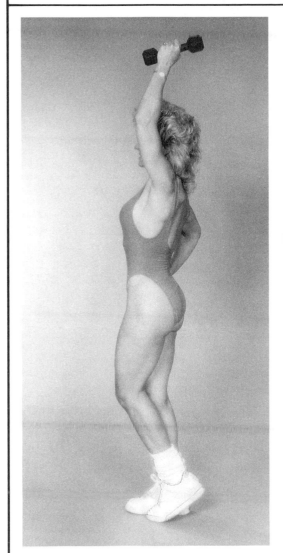

Start

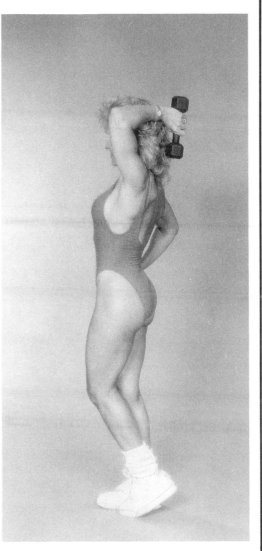

Finish

2. One-Arm Triceps Kickback

This exercise develops and shapes the entire triceps muscle.

START: Stand with your feet together, bending at the waist and at the knees. Holding a dumbbell in your right hand, with your palm facing your body, bend your right arm at the elbow so that your right upper arm is nearly parallel to your body and your elbow is touching your waist.

ACTION: Keeping your upper arm close to your body, extend your right arm back as far as possible. As you reach the farthest point, flex your triceps muscle as hard as possible. Return to the start position and repeat the movement until you have completed your set. Repeat the set for your left arm then, without resting, begin the first set of your next triceps exercise, the flat cross-face triceps extension.

ATTENTION: It is crucial that you keep your upper arm close to your body throughout the exercise.

ALTERNATIVES: You may perform this exercise by leaning on a flat exercise bench with one knee. You may do this exercise with two arms at a time.

ONE-ARM TRICEPS KICKBACK

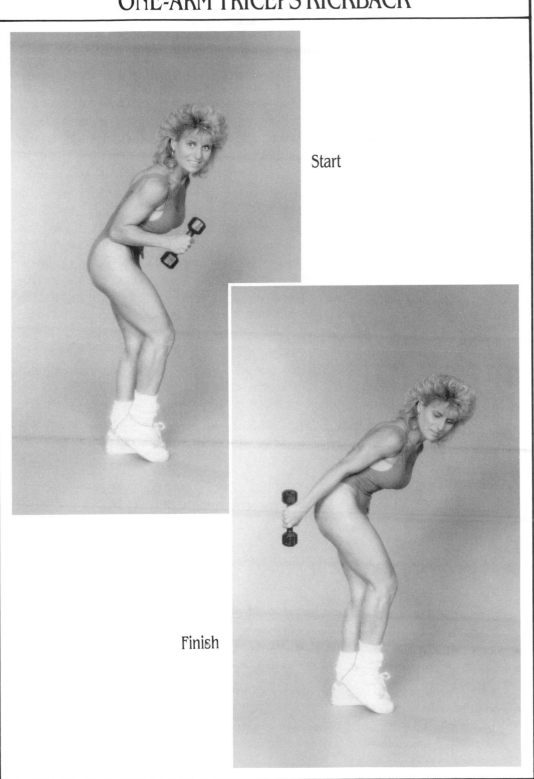

Start

Finish

3. Flat Cross-Face Triceps Extension

This exercise develops and shapes the inner head of the triceps muscle.

START: Lie on a flat exercise bench with a dumbbell held in your fully extended right arm, with your palm facing your body. To avoid hitting yourself in the face, avert your face as you move the dumbbell.

ACTION: Bending your right arm at the elbow, lower your arm until the dumbbell touches your left neck-shoulder area. Return to the start position and repeat the movement until you have completed your set. Repeat the set for the left arm. If you are using the regular Fat-Burning Workout, take a ten- to fifteen-second rest before beginning the second set of your first triceps exercise. If not, proceed to the next triceps exercise, the incline cross-face triceps extension, without resting.

ATTENTION: Remember to flex your triceps on the down movement and to feel the stretch in that muscle on the up movement. Do not let your upper arm wander away from the close-to-the-head position. Strict form is crucial in this and all other exercises.

4. Incline Cross-face Triceps Extension

(for Intensity and Insanity workouts)

This exercise develops and shapes the entire triceps muscle. Follow the instructions for the previous exercise, only do this exercise on an incline bench.

When you complete this exercise you may rest ten to fifteen seconds before beginning the second set of your first triceps exercise.

FLAT CROSS-FACE TRICEPS EXTENSION

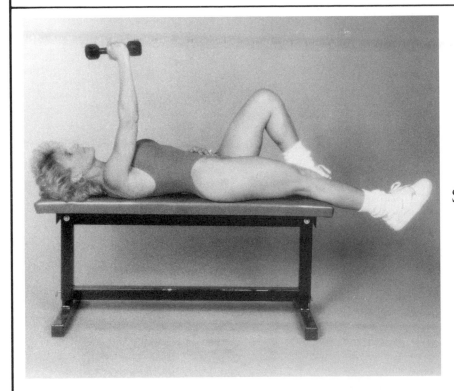

Start

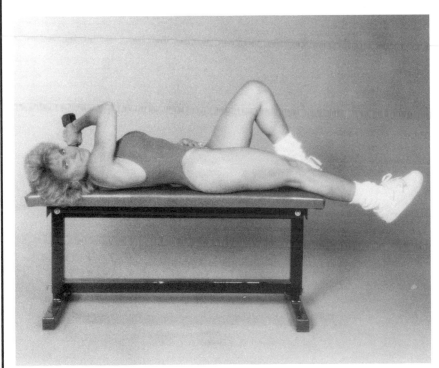

Finish

BACK ROUTINE

1. Reverse Bent Dumbbell Row

This exercise develops and shapes the lats and trapezius muscles.

START: Stand with your feet a natural width apart, holding a dumbbell in each hand, your palms facing away from your body. Arching your back, bend forward until your torso is almost parallel to the ground. Hold the dumbbells about six inches away from your body, and in line with either knee.

ACTION: Keeping your mind on your latissimus dorsi muscles, raise the dumbbells until they reach waist height, but keep them the same six inches away from the sides of your body. Flex your latissimus dorsi muscles and return to the start position. Stretch your latissimus dorsi muscles and repeat the movement until you have completed your set. Without resting, do your first set of the next exercise, the bent dumbbell shrug.

ATTENTION: Keep your torso parallel to the floor. Be sure to keep the dumbbells six inches away from your body. Imagine that the dumbbells are a barbell. This will help you to maintain the position.

ALTERNATIVES: You may do this exercise with a barbell.

REVERSE BENT DUMBBELL ROW

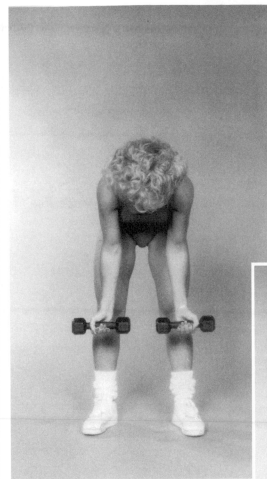

Start

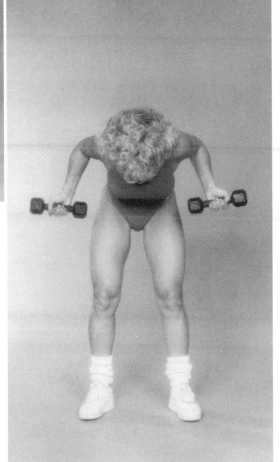

Finish

2. Bent Dumbbell Shrug

This exercise shapes and develops the upper latissimus dorsi muscles and the trapezius muscles.

START: Holding a dumbbell in each hand, with your palms facing your body, bend at the waist until your torso is nearly parallel to the floor. Your arms should be straight down and in front of your knees.

ACTION: Unbending at the waist, rise to an upright position, but as you go along, raise your shoulders as high as possible and when you reach the standing up position, shrug your shoulders back and down. Return to the start position and repeat the movement until you have completed your set. Without resting, begin the first set of your next back exercise, the dumbbell upright row.

ATTENTION: This exercise is not just a shrug. It's a latissimus dorsi expansion exercise as well. Each time you rise to standing position, be sure to feel the stretch in your upper lat muscles as well as in your trapezius muscles.

BENT DUMBBELL SHRUG

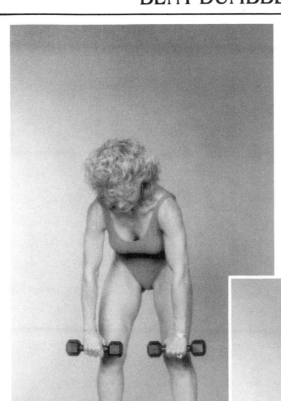

Start

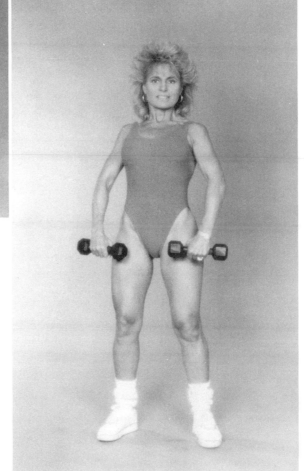

Finish

3. Dumbbell Upright Row

This exercise develops and shapes the entire trapezius muscle. It also strengthens the front deltoid muscle.

START: Stand with your feet a natural width apart and hold a dumbbell with both hands in the center, your palms facing your body.

ACTION: Extending your elbows outward and keeping the dumbbell close to your body, raise the dumbbell until it reaches chin height. Flex your shoulder and trapezius muscles and return to the start position. Repeat the movement until you have completed your set. If you are following the regular Fat-Burning Workout, you may take a ten- to fifteen-second rest before beginning the second set of your first back exercise. If not, immediately proceed to the first set of your next back exercise, the seated dumbbell back lateral.

ATTENTION: Maintain a fluid movement throughout this exercise. Do not yield to the temptation to rest between repetitions. If you are having trouble performing the exercise, go to a lighter weight. Form and consistency are more important than the weight you are using.

ALTERNATIVES: You may use a barbell to perform this exercise. Grasp the barbell with your thumbs about six to eight inches apart.

DUMBBELL UPRIGHT ROW

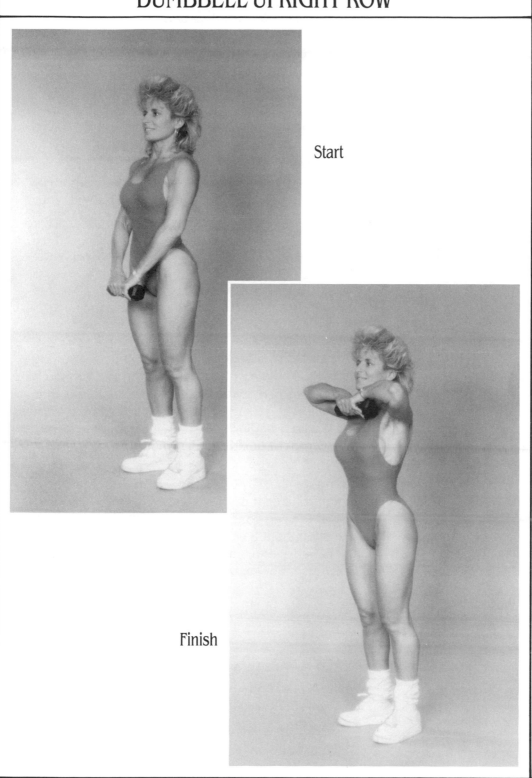

Start

Finish

4. Seated Dumbbell Back Lateral

(for Intensity and Insanity workouts)

This exercise develops, shapes, and defines the upper back and trapezius muscles.

START: While holding a dumbbell in each hand, sit at the edge of a flat exercise bench and lean forward until your upper body is nearly parallel to the floor. Hold the dumbbells with your palms facing away from you behind your ankles. Let the ends of the dumbbells touch each other.

ACTION: Keeping them close to your legs at all times, raise the dumbbells up and back, rotating the dumbbells as you go along so that when you reach hip level your palms are facing away from your body and either side of each dumbbell is about 3–4 inches from your hip area. Return to the start position and repeat the movement until you have completed your set. If you are following the Intensity Fat-Burning Workout, you may rest for ten to fifteen seconds before beginning the second set of your first back exercise. If you are following the Insanity Fat-Burning Workout, begin the first set of your next exercise, the lying dumbbell back lateral, without resting.

ATTENTION: Flex your upper back muscles on the up movement and allow them to stretch out fully on the down movement. Remember to keep your arms as close to your sides as possible throughout the exercise. Don't hold your breath. Breathe naturally and work in a steady, deliberate manner. Don't rush, but keep moving.

ALTERNATIVES: For this exercise you may substitute the pulley row, which can be done on any gym rowing machine.

SEATED DUMBBELL BACK LATERAL

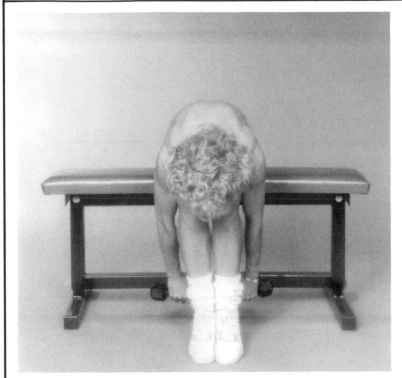

Start

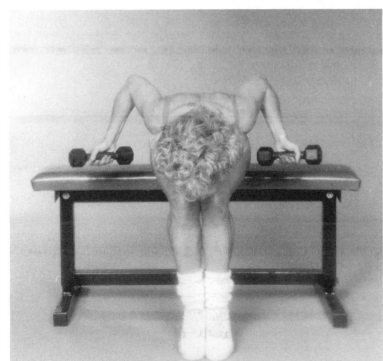

Finish

5. Lying Dumbbell Back Lateral

(for Insanity workouts)

This exercise develops and shapes the latissimus dorsi muscles and helps to define the upper back muscles.

START: Lie face downward on a flat exercise bench with a dumbbell held in each hand and palms facing your body.

ACTION: Bending at the elbows and keeping your arms as close to the bench and your body as possible, raise the dumb-bells until you cannot bend your arms any farther. Flex your latissimus dorsi muscles and squeeze your back. Return to the start position. Feel the stretch in your latissimus dorsi muscles. Repeat the movement until you have completed your set. Rest for ten to fifteen seconds and then begin the second set of your first back exercise.

ATTENTION: If you are a large-breasted woman, you may find this exercise a bit awkward at first. Place a pillow under your breast area for comfort.

ALTERNATIVES: You may substitute the lat pull-down to the front on any gym lat pull-down machine for this exercise.

LYING DUMBBELL BACK LATERAL

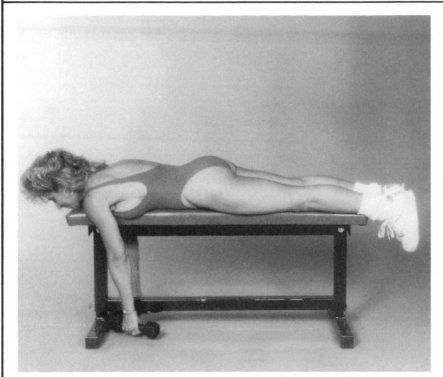

Start

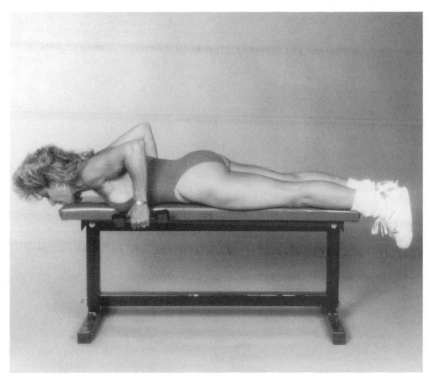

Finish

REVIEW OF EXERCISES CONTAINED IN THIS CHAPTER

Biceps

1. Standing alternate dumbbell curl
2. Standing angled simultaneous dumbbell curl
3. Standing alternate hammer curl
4. Concentration curl

Chest

1. Incline dumbbell press
2. Incline dumbbell flye with a twist
3. Cross-bench pullover
4. Flat dumbbell flye
5. Flat dumbbell press

Shoulders

1. Standing side lateral
2. Standing front lateral
3. Pee-wee lateral
4. Bent lateral
5. Standing alternate dumbbell press

Triceps

1. One-arm overhead triceps extension
2. One-arm triceps kickback
3. Flat cross-face triceps extension
4. Incline cross-face triceps extension

Back

1. Reverse bent dumbbell row
2. Bent dumbbell shrug
3. Dumbbell upright row
4. Seated dumbbell back lateral
5. Lying dumbbell back lateral

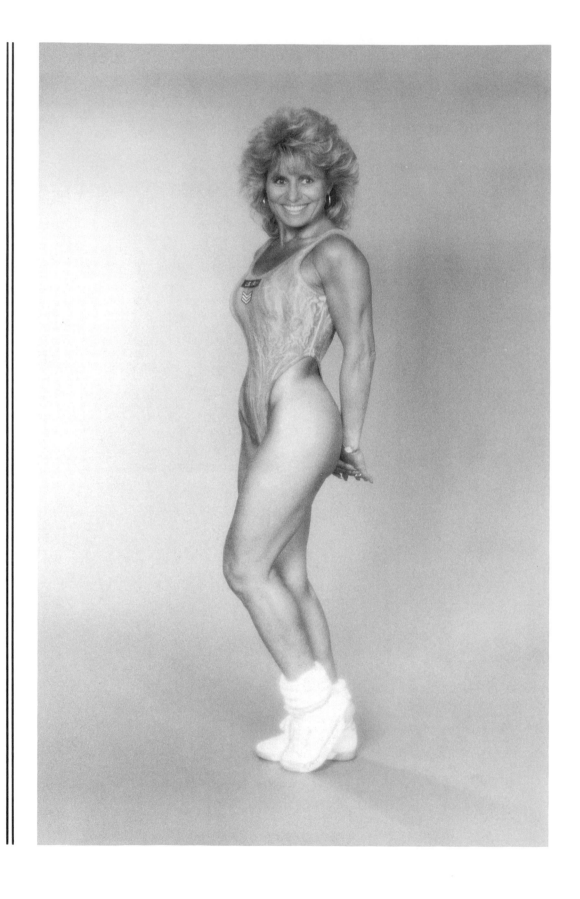

7 | THE LOWER BODY WORKOUT

This chapter contains the lower body workout. You will do this workout on alternate exercise days. As with the upper body routine, if you choose the regular Fat-Burning Workout, you will do only the first three exercises listed for each body part. If you choose the Intensity Fat-Burning Workout, you will do the first four exercises listed for each body part, and if you choose the Insanity Fat-Burning Workout, you will do *all* exercises presented in this chapter.

WHY EXERCISE THE BODY PARTS
IN THIS PARTICULAR ORDER?

The body parts exercised in this chapter are: thighs, hip-buttocks, abdominals, and calves. Your thighs are composed of powerful muscles—your quadriceps (located on your front thighs) and your biceps femoris (located on your back thighs). Because these muscles are so strong, it is a good idea to exercise them first. You will feel empowered two minutes into the workout, and this feeling of power will serve as a catalyst to stir up your energy for the rest of the grueling lower body workout.

Because your hips and buttocks are directly connected to your thighs (your side-front thighs are connected to your hips, and your back thighs are connected to your buttocks), it makes sense to exercise them next, in order to completely exhaust this muscle group. (You will notice that many of the thigh and hip-buttock exercises overlap in the muscle groups that they challenge.)

The abdominal muscles are exercised after your hip-buttocks area, because we don't want to leave them for last. Working them effectively requires a lot of energy. (Yet we don't want to exercise them first because one really needs to warm up with less tedious exercises before beginning the challenging abdominal workout.)

Calves are exercised last because they are the most easily exercised muscle group in the lower body workout. Exercising calves last can serve as the carrot on the stick during your workout. For example, in the middle of your abdominal workout, you may be feeling tired and may even be thinking of not completing your workout. Then you will realize that after you finish the abdominal muscles, all you have to do is work your calves. It's clear sailing. So chances are, you will bite the bullet and complete your abdominals, then relax and do your calves without too much effort. The end result? You will have psyched yourself into finishing your workout, and you will rightfully be proud of yourself.

WHY DO THE EXERCISES FOR EACH BODY PART IN THE ORDER GIVEN?

I have carefully placed the exercises for each body part in a certain order so that you will be able to move from one exercise to the next with the least waste of time.

You will note that most of the time there is no need to change position at all for the first three exercises. This means that if you are following the regular Fat-Burning Workout, you will have very little moving about to do. If you are following the Intensity or Insanity Fat-Burning Workout, sometimes you will have to change position slightly. But in this case, you can always opt for the speed set.

AN IMPORTANT REMINDER ABOUT EXERCISING BUTTOCKS AND ABDOMINALS

You will not be using the modified pyramid system when you exercise your buttocks and abdominals. Instead, you will do all sets with little or no weight (see the specific exercise descriptions). You will always do from fifteen to twenty-five repetitions of each set of these exercises. Of course, you will only do as many repetitions per set as you can in the beginning—even if that means only three or four repetitions. In time, you will build up to the required amount. Remember, there is no rush. As long as you put in real effort to complete as many repetitions as you can, you are working hard enough.

120

THIGH ROUTINE

1. Regular Squat

This exercise develops and shapes the front thigh (quadriceps) muscle, and helps to tighten and tone the buttocks (gluteus maximus).

START: With a dumbbell held in each hand, stand with your feet about eight inches apart and your toes slightly pointed outward. Let your arms hang down at your sides, holding the dumbbells with your palms facing your body. Keep your back straight and your eyes looking straight ahead.

ACTION: Rising slightly on your toes if necessary, descend to a squatting position. The goal is to get a 45-degree bend in your knees, but if you cannot get that low, don't worry about it. Feel the stretch in your quadriceps muscles and return to the start position. Flex your quadriceps and buttocks muscles and repeat the movement until you have completed your set. Without resting, proceed to your next exercise, the lunge.

ATTENTION: Maintain a fluid movement. Avoid bouncing back up off your knees. Keep the pressure on your front thigh muscles. Make them do the work. Don't lean forward or rock your body. If you keep your eyes straight ahead, you will find it easier to maintain your balance.

ALTERNATIVES: You may place a two-by-four piece of wood under your heels if you feel it helps you with balance. You may use a barbell, placed across your shoulders behind your neck, instead of dumbbells.

REGULAR SQUAT

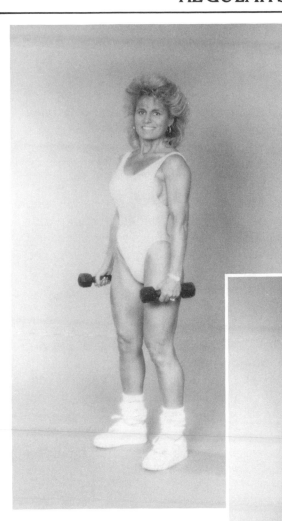

Start

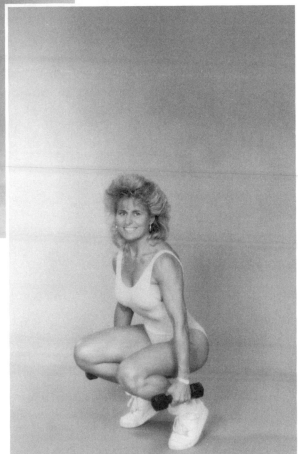

Finish

2. Lunge

This exercise develops and shapes the front thigh (quadriceps) muscle. It also helps to tighten and tone the hip-buttocks area.

START: Stand with your feet a natural width apart and your back straight. Hold a dumbbell in each hand, with your palms facing your body and your arms straight down at your sides. Look straight ahead.

ACTION: Step forward about two and a half feet with your left foot, or until you cannot "lunge" any farther, bending your right knee as you go. Return to the start position and repeat the movement until you have completed your set. Repeat the set for your other leg then, without resting, proceed to your next exercise, the sissy squat.

ATTENTION: In order to keep your balance, avoid looking down at your legs. Instead, look straight ahead of you. Do not bounce back up off the non-lunging leg. Stretch your extended back leg, and feel the flex in your bent leg with each repetition. Without resting, proceed to your next thigh exercise, the sissy squat.

ALTERNATIVES: You may use a barbell, placed across your shoulders behind your neck, instead of dumbbells.

LUNGE

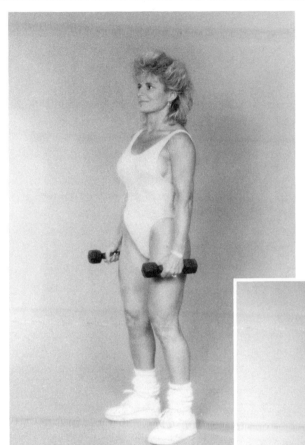

Start

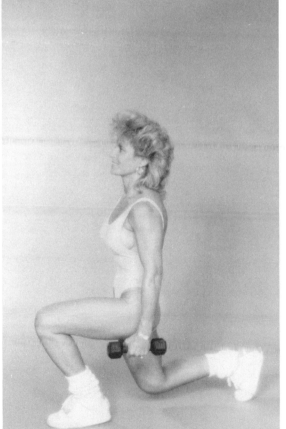

Finish

3. Sissy Squat

This exercise develops, shapes, and gives definition to the front thigh (quadriceps) muscle. It also helps to tighten and tone the hip-buttocks area.

START: Stand with your feet about five inches apart and your toes pointed slightly outward. Place your right hand on a stable object, such as a post, high bench, bar, or railing.

ACTION: Raise yourself up on your toes and, at the same time, lean your upper body back as far as you can and feel a full stretch in your quadriceps muscles. At the same time, squeeze your buttocks as hard as possible. You will be completely up on your toes at this point. Keep your hips in line with your ankles as you work. Return to the start position and repeat the movement until you have completed your set. If you are performing the regular Fat-Burning Workout, you may rest for ten to fifteen seconds before beginning the next set of your first thigh exercise. If you are performing the Intensity or Insanity Fat-Burning Workout, proceed to the next exercise, the front squat.

ATTENTION: In the case of this exercise, a picture is worth a thousand words. Look at the photograph and follow it.

ALTERNATIVES: You may perform this exercise with no weight on a machine, or with a light weight on a lying leg press machine (you will be in a lying position).

SISSY SQUAT

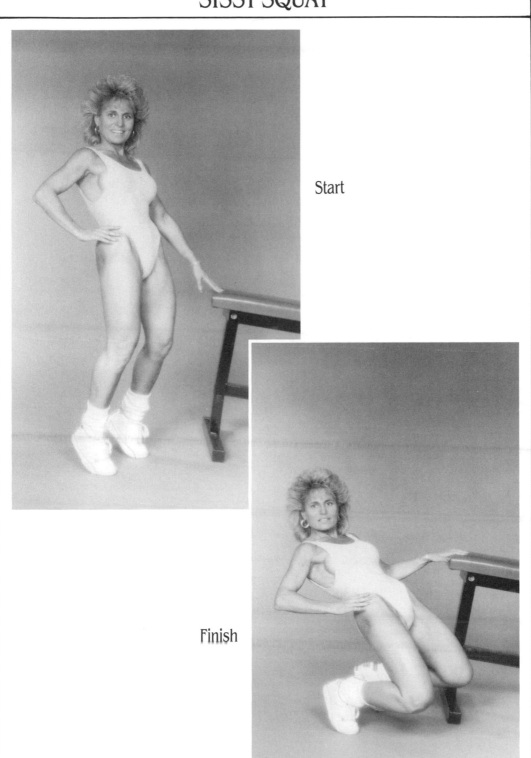

Start

Finish

126

4. Front Squat

(for Intensity and Insanity workouts)

This exercise develops, shapes, and gives definition to the front thigh muscle (quadriceps).

START: Stand with your feet a natural width apart, with your toes angled out slightly. Hold a dumbbell in each hand, and cross your arms in front of your chest. The ends of the dumbbells will be touching your shoulders. Look straight ahead and keep your back straight.

ACTION: Keeping your upper body straight and rising up on your toes if necessary, descend into the squat position until you cannot descend any farther. Feel a full stretch in your quadriceps muscles and return to start. Flex your quadriceps muscles and repeat the movement until you have completed your set. If you are performing the Intensity Fat-Burning Workout, you may rest for ten to fifteen seconds before beginning the next set of your first thigh exercise. If you are performing the Insanity Fat-Burning Workout, proceed to your next thigh exercise, the leg curl, without resting.

ATTENTION: Beware the temptation to bounce up off the balls of your feet when rising from the squat position. Force your quadriceps to do the work instead.

ALTERNATIVES: You may hold a barbell instead of dumbbells above your crossed arms. You may place a two-by-four board under your heels if you feel that you need it for balance.

If you are working out in a gym, you may substitute the leg press, done on any leg press machine, for this exercise.

FRONT SQUAT

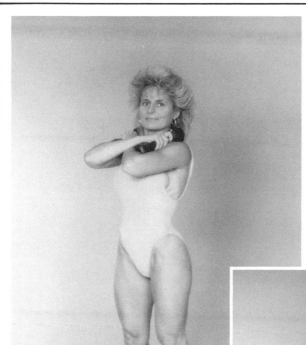

Start

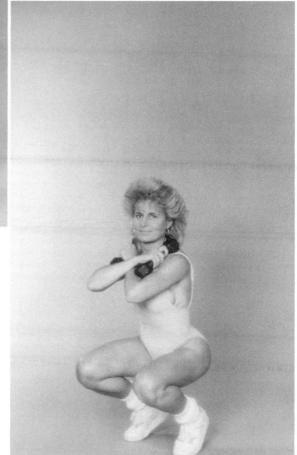

Finish

5. Leg Curl

(for the Insanity Workout)

This exercise develops, shapes, and gives definition to the back thigh (biceps femoris, or hamstrings) muscle.

START: With a dumbbell placed between your feet, lie facedown on a flat exercise bench. Extend your legs straight out behind you and lean on your elbows for support.

ACTION: Keeping your feet together to hold the dumbbell in place, and bending at the knees, raise your lower legs until they are perpendicular to the floor. Flex your back thigh muscles and return to start position. Feel the stretch in your back thigh muscles and repeat the movement until you have completed your set. You may rest for ten to fifteen seconds before beginning the next set of your first thigh exercise.

ATTENTION: Beware of the temptation to swing the dumbbell up and down. Keep your movements deliberate by consciously flexing on the up movement and stretching on the down movement. Keep your abdominal area glued to the bench.

ALTERNATIVES: If you are at a gym, you may perform this exercise on any leg curl machine.

LEG CURL

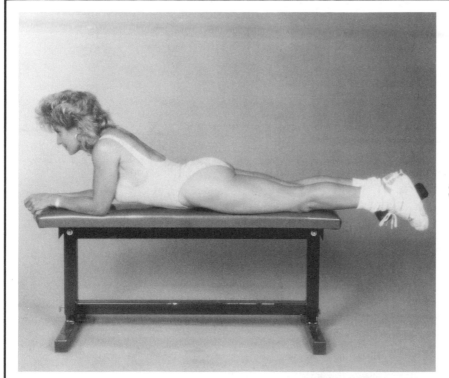

Start

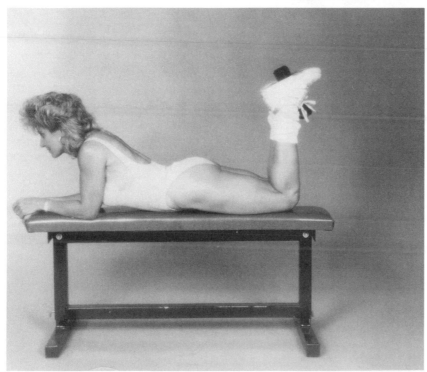

Finish

BUTTOCKS ROUTINE

1. One-Legged Butt Lift

This exercise tightens and tones the entire hip-buttocks area.

START: Face an object you can hold for support, such as a bench. Kneel with your back straight and your shoulders slightly forward. Extend your left arm fully as you grasp the supporting object.

ACTION: Point your toes behind you and raise your right knee to the side and extend your leg behind you, all the time squeezing your right hip-buttock as hard as possible. (Your knee will be about eight inches off the floor in its final position.) Continuing to keep the pressure on your right hip-buttock area, return to the start position and repeat the movement until you have completed your set. Immediately perform the set for the other side of your body. Then, without resting, proceed to your next hip-buttocks exercise, the lying butt lift.

ATTENTION: Do not arch your back. Keep it straight throughout the movement. Keep your shoulders forward. It is okay to lean slightly to the side opposite your working leg.

ALTERNATIVES: Instead of moving your leg to the side and slightly back, you may extend your leg straight out behind you until your knee is locked, all the time squeezing your working buttock.

ONE-LEGGED BUTT LIFT

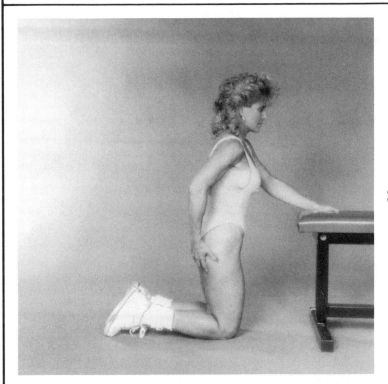

Start

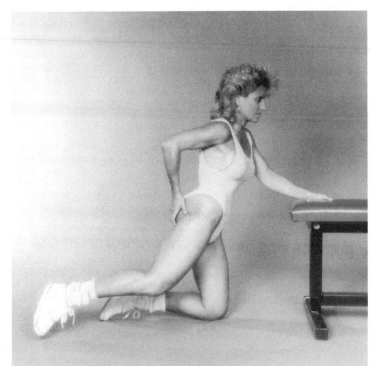

Finish

2. Lying Butt Lift

This exercise tightens and tones the entire hip-buttocks area. In addition, it helps to tone the biceps femoris (back thigh) and to strengthen the lower back.

START: Lie flat on your back on the floor and bend your knees until your feet are about eight inches apart and flat on the floor. Place your hands, palms up, just under your lower buttocks area.

ACTION: Squeezing your entire hip-buttocks area as hard as you can, raise yourself to the highest position possible. As you reach the peak position, flex your entire buttocks as hard as you can, giving your lower buttocks an extra hard flex, and all the time keeping your hands on your working buttocks muscles so you can tell how much of a flex you are getting. Return to the start position and repeat the movement until you have completed your set. Without resting, proceed to your next hip-buttocks exercise, the feather kick-up.

ATTENTION: This is a very effective exercise *if* you give it everything you've got. It is especially important to make an additional effort to flex the lower buttocks area by lifting a little higher just when you are tempted to say, "Enough."

LYING BUTT LIFT

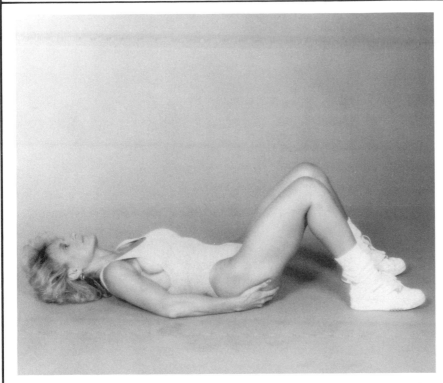

Start

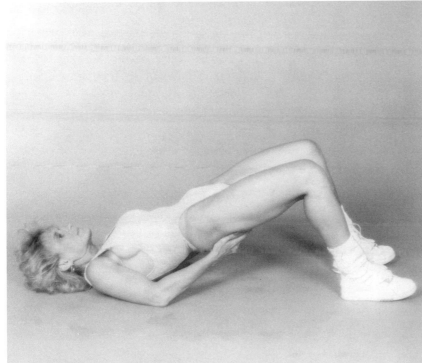

Finish

3. Feather Kick-Up

This exercise tightens and tones the entire hip-buttocks area. It also helps to firm the biceps femoris (back thigh).

START: Get on the floor on all fours. Raise your left thigh up and bend at the knee so that your leg takes the shape of an "L."

ACTION: Pointing your toe behind you, straighten your left leg by raising it and unbending your knee at the same time. Continue this movement until you cannot raise your leg any higher. Flex your buttocks and return to the start position and repeat the movement until you have completed your set. Immediately do the set for the other leg. You must apply continual tension to your working buttocks muscles, both on the up and down movement. If you are performing the regular Fat-Burning Workout, you may rest for ten to fifteen seconds before beginning the next set of your first hip-buttocks exercise. If you are performing the Intensity or Insanity workout, proceed to your next hip-buttocks exercise, the prone butt lift.

ATTENTION: It is crucial that you return to the "L" position each time you unbend your leg. Although this exercise takes a few weeks to get used to, it is well worth the trouble. It is one of the most effective butt lifters available.

FEATHER KICK-UP

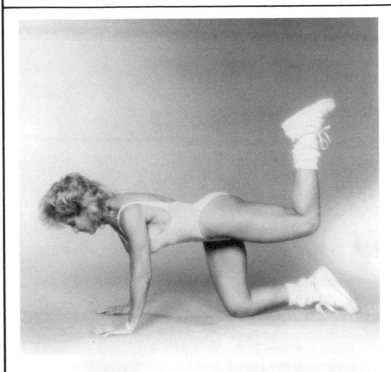

Start

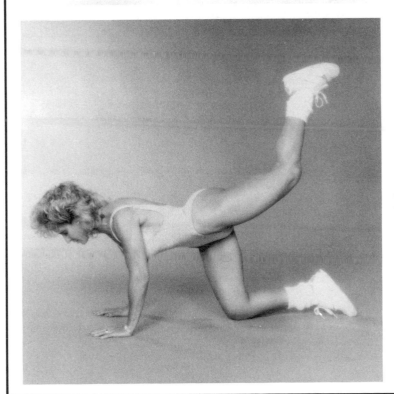

Finish

4. Prone Butt Lift

(for Intensity and Insanity workouts)

This exercise tightens and tones the entire hip-buttocks area. In addition, it helps to tone the biceps femoris (back thigh) and to strengthen the lower back.

START: Lie on the floor on your stomach. Lean on your elbows for support. Extend your toes behind you.

ACTION: Squeezing your entire hip-buttocks area as hard as possible and keeping your knees locked, lift both legs at the same time until you cannot go any higher. Your legs will naturally go into a wider position at this point (about twelve inches apart). Now give your hip-buttocks area an extra hard flex. Keeping the pressure on, return to the start position, and repeat the movement until you have completed your set. If you are performing the Intensity Fat-Burning Workout, you may rest for ten to fifteen seconds before beginning the next set of your first hip-buttocks exercise. If you are performing the Insanity Fat-Burning Workout, proceed to your next hip-buttocks exercise, the scissors, without resting.

ATTENTION: Relax your lower back. Don't allow it to tense as you work.

ALTERNATIVES: You may perform this exercise one leg at a time.

PRONE BUTT LIFT

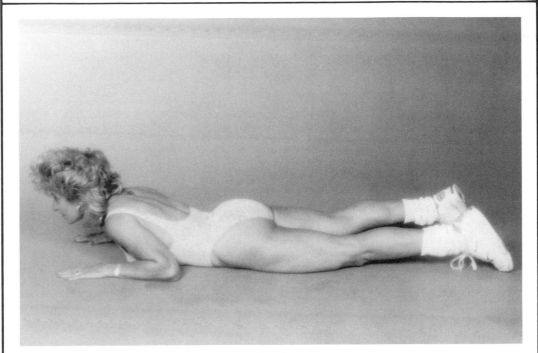

Start

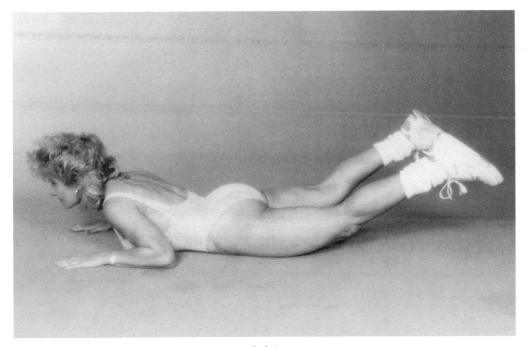

Finish

5. Scissors

(for the Insanity workout)

This exercise tightens and tones the entire hip-buttocks area. It also helps to firm the front thigh (quadriceps) muscle.

START: Sit at the edge of a flat exercise bench and place your hands, palms facing down, under each buttock. Extend your legs straight out in front of you until your knees are locked. Point your toes forward.

ACTION: Squeezing your hip-buttocks area as hard as possible, scissor your legs apart until you cannot go any farther. You should be able to feel the complete flexing of your buttocks with your hands. Continuing to squeeze as hard as possible, return to the start position. Repeat the movement until you have completed your set. You may rest for ten to fifteen seconds before beginning the next set of your first hip-buttocks exercise.

ATTENTION: This is one of the most enjoyable and relaxing hip-buttocks exercises available, yet it is highly effective. Take advantage of this and try to do as many repetitions as possible, all the time squeezing your hip-buttocks area as hard as possible.

ALTERNATIVES: You may do this exercise with light ankle weights (one to three pounds).

SCISSORS

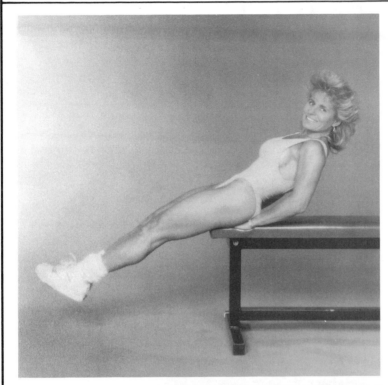

Start

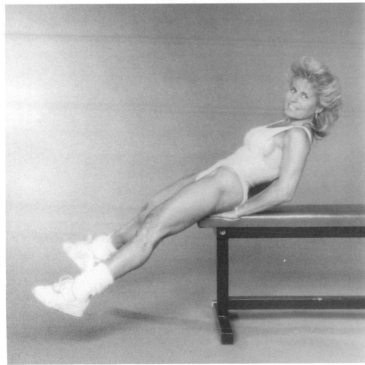

Finish

140

ABDOMINAL ROUTINE

1. Sit-up

This exercise tightens and tones the upper abdominal area. It also helps to strengthen the lower back.

START: Lie on the floor, flat on your back, and bend your knees to a 30-degree angle. Place your hands behind your neck, or cross them in front of you on your chest.

ACTION: Flexing your upper abdominal muscles as hard as possible, raise yourself off the floor until you are sitting up. (The movement is one of curling rather than jerking.) Keeping the pressure on your upper abdominal muscles, return to the starting position. Repeat the movement until you have completed your set. Without resting, proceed to your next abdominal exercise, the leg raise.

ATTENTION: Maintain continuous motion. Do not lurch up off the floor or flop back down to start.

ALTERNATIVES: You may perform this exercise with a three- to ten-pound dumbbell held in the center of your upper abdominal area.

SIT-UP

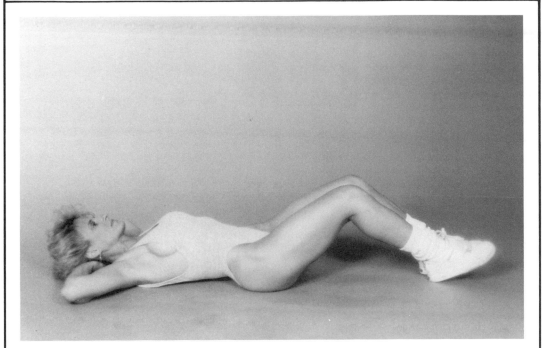

Start

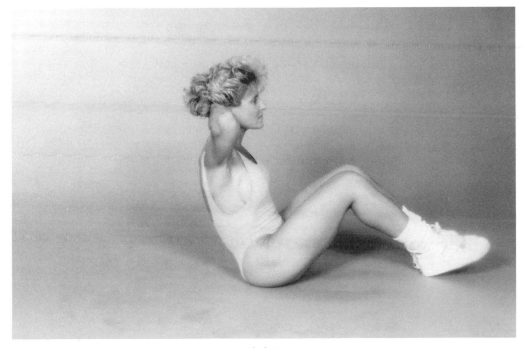

Finish

2. Leg Raise

This exercise tightens and tones the entire lower abdominal area. It also helps to strengthen the lower back.

START: Lie on the floor or a bench, flat on your back, with your arms behind your neck or holding the sides of the bench and your legs extended straight out. Keep your shoulders on the floor or bench, and bend your knees very slightly.

ACTION: Flexing your lower abdominal muscles as hard as possible, raise your legs until they are perpendicular to the floor. Continue to keep the pressure on your lower abdominal muscles as you return to the start position. Repeat the movement until you have completed your set then, without resting, proceed to your next abdominal exercise, the lying leg-in.

ATTENTION: Do not arch your back. Keep it flat on the floor or bench. Beware of the temptation to bounce your legs up from the start position. Maintain fluid movements.

ALTERNATIVES: You may perform this exercise with a three- to ten-pound dumbbell between your feet, or you may use ankle weights.

LEG RAISE

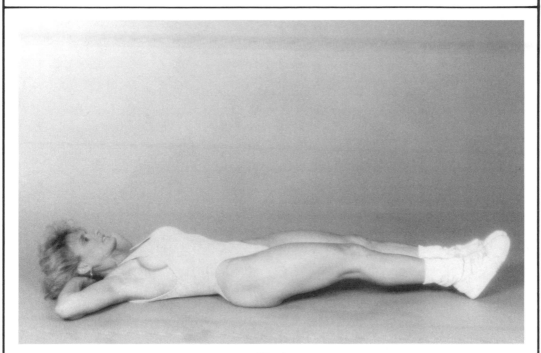

Start

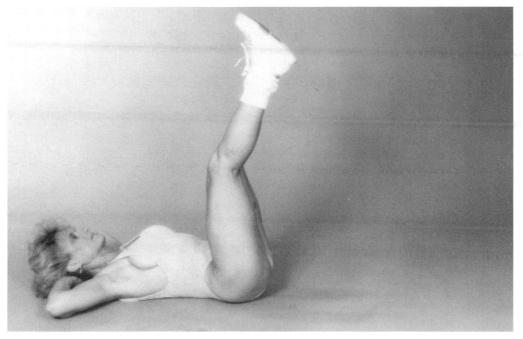

Finish

3. Lying Leg-in

This exercise tightens and tones the entire lower abdominal area. It also helps to strengthen the lower back.

START: Lie on a flat exercise bench so that your buttocks just touch the edge of the bench. Hold onto the bench on either side of you, and extend your legs straight out in front of you. The small of your back should remain flat against the bench at all times, but you may raise your head and neck.

ACTION: Flexing your lower abdominal muscles as hard as possible, pull your knees toward your chest until you cannot go any farther. Keeping the pressure on your lower abdominal muscles, return to the start position and repeat the movement until you have completed your set. If you are performing the regular Fat-Burning Workout, you may rest ten to fifteen seconds before beginning the next set of your first abdominal exercise. If you are performing the Intensity or Insanity Fat-Burning Workout, proceed to your next abdominal exercise, the crunch, without resting.

ATTENTION: Keep your mind on your lower abdominal muscles throughout the exercise. Do not rest between repetitions.

ALTERNATIVES: You may perform this exercise sitting at the edge of an exercise bench, and leaning slightly back. You may place a three- to ten-pound dumbbell between your feet. You may perform this exercise on any pulley machine by using a looped rope—set the weight to about ten pounds. Eventually, you may set it as high as thirty pounds, depending upon how strong your abdominal muscles grow.

LYING LEG-IN

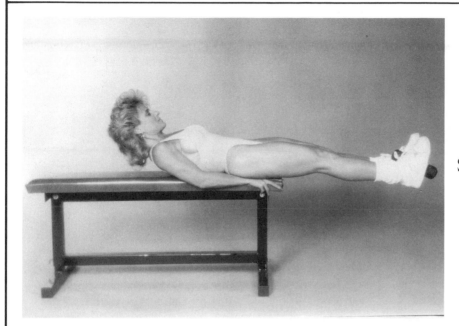

Start

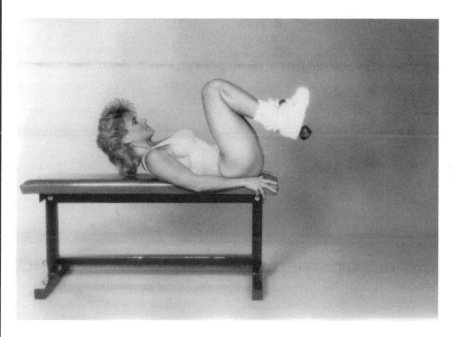

Finish

4. Crunch

(for Intensity and Insanity workouts)

This exercise tightens and tones the entire upper abdominal area. It also helps to strengthen the lower back.

START: Lie flat on your back on the floor, and place your calves over a flat exercise bench. Place your hands behind your neck.

ACTION: Curl your body upward until your shoulders are completely off the ground, all the time flexing your upper abdominal muscles as hard as possible. Without letting up on the tension, return to the start position and repeat the movement until you have finished your set. If you are performing the Intensity Fat-Burning Workout, you may rest ten to fifteen seconds before beginning the next set of your first abdominal exercise. If you are performing the Insanity Fat-Burning Workout, without resting proceed to your next abdominal exercise, the standing serratus crunch.

ATTENTION: This is not a sit-up. You must not raise more than your shoulders off the floor.

ALTERNATIVES: You may perform this exercise by twisting your body from side to side.

CRUNCH

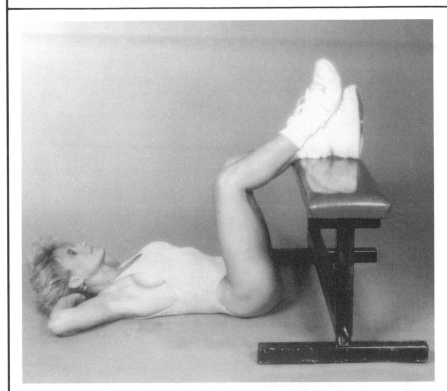

Start

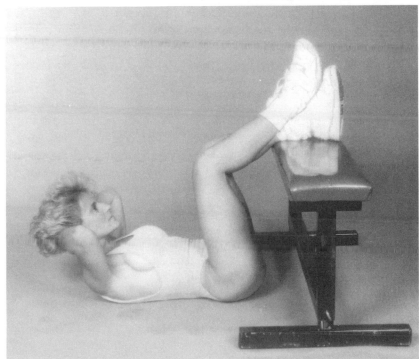

Finish

5. Standing Serratus Crunch

(for Insanity workouts)

This exercise tightens, tones, strengthens, and gives definition to the upper abdominal muscles, especially the side-upper abdominals.

START: Stand with your feet together and with a three-pound dumbbell in your right hand, your palm facing your body. Extend your arm upward and bend your elbow into a slightly rounded "L" position.

ACTION: Bending at the waist and squeezing your right serratus and oblique muscles as hard as possible, lower your elbow and at the same time bend at the waist until you cannot "crunch" any more. Return to the start position and repeat the movement until you have completed your set. Repeat the set for your other arm. You may rest for ten to fifteen seconds before beginning the next set of your first abdominal exercise.

ATTENTION: This is a wonderful exercise. It has been the secret of champion bodybuilders for years. The crucial element is to make sure that you are doing the work with your serratus and oblique muscles and not with your arm. For this reason, you must never go higher than a three-pound dumbbell.

ALTERNATIVES: You may perform this exercise on any pulley machine, including the lat pull-down machine pulley. In this case, you will use a looped rope. If one is not available, you may use a narrow bar and intertwine your fingers around the center of the bar. You may also use a triangle device usually used for cable crossovers. When performing this exercise on the pulley machine, you will need to set the weight at ten pounds. Eventually your abdominal muscles may become strong enough to need a twenty-pound challenge.

STANDING SERRATUS CRUNCH

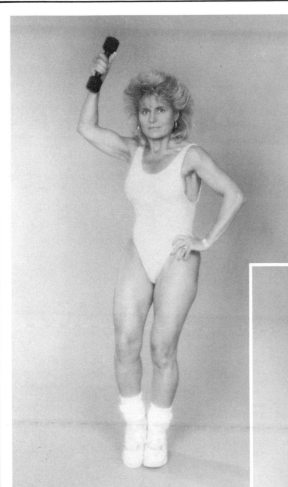

Start

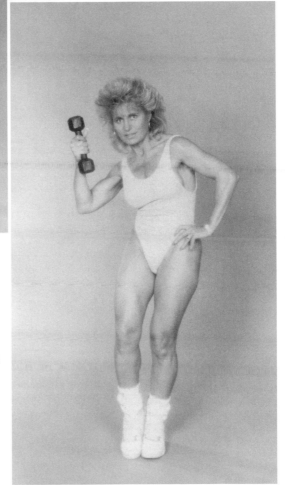

Finish

CALF ROUTINE

1. Seated Straight-Toe Calf Raise

This exercise develops and shapes the entire gastrocnemius (calf) muscle.

START: Sit on the edge of a flat exercise bench, with a dumbbell held between your knees and your toes on a thick book or four-inch block of wood. Bend forward, and lower your heels as close to the ground as possible.

ACTION: Keeping your toes pointed straight ahead, raise your heels as high as possible. When you reach the high point, flex your calf muscles as hard as possible and return to the start position, letting your calf muscles stretch out to the fullest extent. Repeat the movement until you have completed your set. Without resting, proceed to your next calf exercise, the seated angled-out-toe calf raise.

ATTENTION: Maintain a fluid movement. Do not bounce up or drop down on your toes.

ALTERNATIVES: You may perform this exercise on any seated calf machine.

2. Seated Angled-Out-Toe Calf Raise

This exercise develops and shapes the entire calf muscle, especially the inner calf area.

Follow the instructions for the seated straight-toe calf raise, only this time angle your toes out to the side (away from your body) as far as you can go.

When you complete your set, proceed at once to your next calf exercise, the seated angled-in-toe calf raise.

3. Seated Angled-in-Toe Calf Raise

This exercise develops and shapes the entire gastrocnemius muscle, especially the outer calf area.

Follow the instructions for the seated straight-toe calf raise, only this time angle your toes inward (your toes should be about four inches apart and angled in to a comfortable position).

If you are performing the regular Fat-Burning Workout, you may take a ten- to fifteen-second break before beginning the next set of your first calf exercise. If you are performing the Intensity or Insanity workout, proceed to your next calf exercise, the standing straight-toe calf raise, without resting.

SEATED STRAIGHT-TOE CALF RAISE

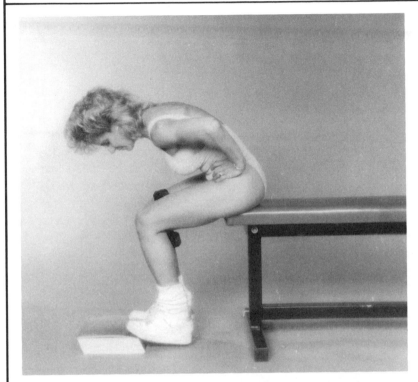

Start

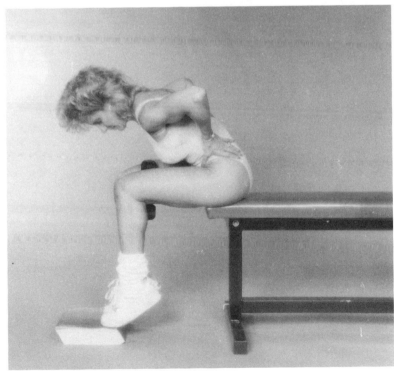

Finish

4. Standing Straight-Toe Calf Raise

(for Intensity and Insanity workouts)

This exercise develops and shapes the entire calf muscle. It also helps to stretch the Achilles tendon.

START: If necessary, stand near an object you can hold for support and on a four-inch-thick book or piece of wood, with a dumbbell in your right hand and the heel and arch of your right foot completely off the book or wood. Raise your left foot up and out of the way. Lower your right heel as close to the ground as possible.

ACTION: Raise yourself onto your right toes as high as possible, and when you reach the high point, flex your calf muscle. Return to the start position and feel the stretch in your calf muscle. Repeat the movement until you have completed your set. Repeat the set for the other leg. You may rest for ten to fifteen seconds before beginning the next set of your first calf exercise.

ATTENTION: Be sure to stretch your calf muscle fully on each down movement. This is also the way you stretch your Achilles tendon.

ALTERNATIVES: You may do this exercise on the edge of a stair. You may perform this exercise on any standing calf machine or leg-press machine.

STANDING STRAIGHT-TOE CALF RAISE

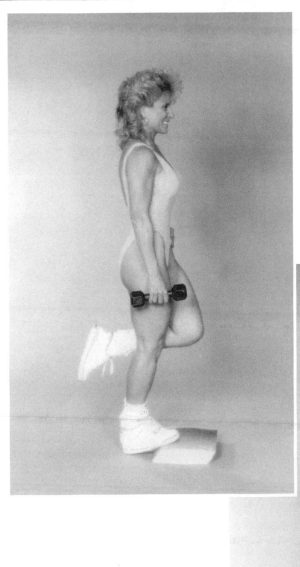

Start

Finish

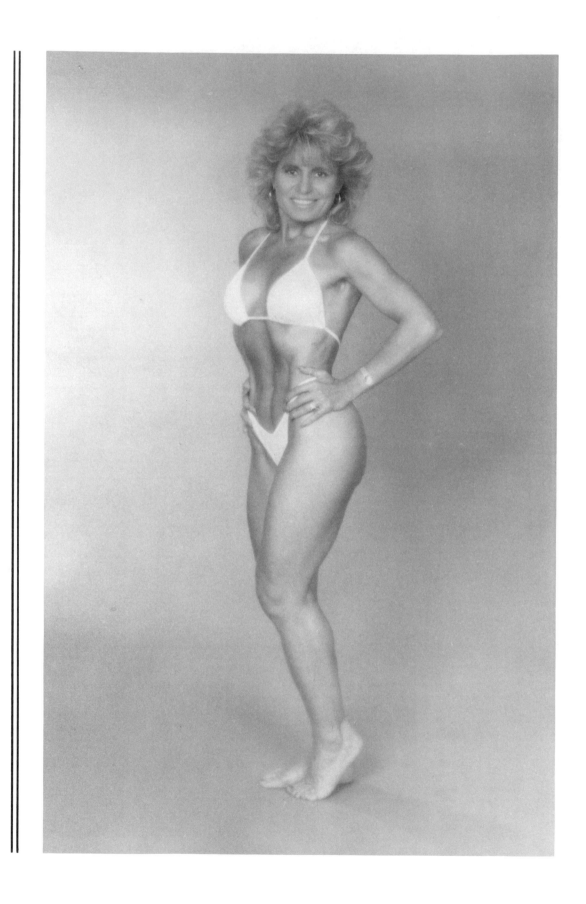

REVIEW OF EXERCISES
CONTAINED IN THIS CHAPTER

Thighs

1. Regular squat
2. Lunge
3. Sissy squat
4. Front squat
5. Leg curl

Buttocks

1. One-legged butt lift
2. Lying butt lift
3. Feather kick-up
4. Prone butt lift
5. Scissors

Abdominals

1. Sit-up
2. Leg raise
3. Lying leg-in
4. Crunch
5. Standing serratus crunch

Calves

1. Seated straight-toe calf raise
2. Seated angled-out toe calf raise
3. Seated angled-in-toe calf raise
4. Standing straight-toe calf raise

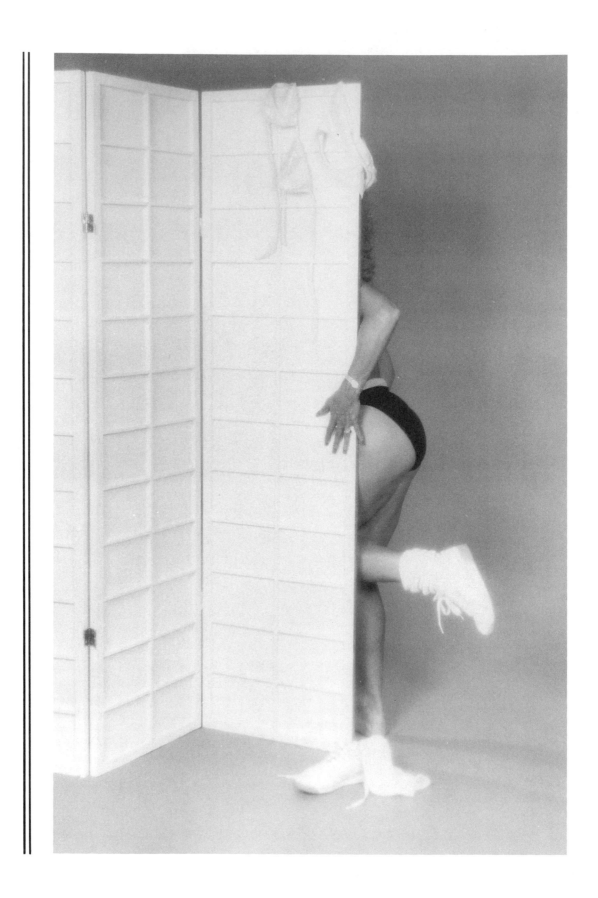

8 | YOU <u>ARE</u> WHAT YOU EAT

We've all heard the expression "You are what you eat." And it's true. If your diet consists of 40 percent fat, as does that of the average American, you are fat—even if you are not overweight. And chances are you feel fat, too, and not just to the touch. You feel sluggish—not as energetic as you would feel if your body were comprised of a higher percentage of muscle.

We've already discussed ways to increase muscle and decrease fat through exercise. Now it's time to talk about the role of diet. If you were to change your eating habits, and cut your fat intake to 20 percent fat, or 20 to 30 grams of fat per day, there would be an amazing difference in your appearance in a matter of months. It is virtually impossible to remain fat if you consistently consume less than 20 percent fat in your diet.

All well and good, but where do you begin? How do you go about correcting a lifetime of poor eating habits? How can you tell which foods to avoid and which to seek out?

In the following paragraphs you will be given simple guidelines on how to avoid fat without ever counting calories. Instead you will focus on the fat content of your food. The only counting you will do will be that of fat grams.

You will also learn which protein foods to eat—and which to avoid because they are also high in fat. You'll find out that sugar is not as bad as everyone seems to think.

STOP FEELING GUILTY ABOUT EATING: CALORIES KEEP YOU ALIVE

If you don't put gas in the car, the motor will not start when you turn the ignition key. Similarly, if you do not put food into your body, nothing will happen when you attempt to move. You will be too weak to get from point A to point B. So it's silly to feel guilty every time you put food in your mouth. The fact is, we must all eat to live.

One of the goals of this chapter is to help you enjoy your food without guilt, and to help you feel in control of your eating so that once you reach your weight goal you can even enjoy "forbidden" foods occasionally.

Food translates into fuel for the body in the form of calories. Technically speaking, a calorie is the amount of energy required to raise the temperature of one gram of water one degree Celsius. In simple terms, the number of calories in a given food item is the amount of energy of fuel available in that particular food item.

FAT CALORIES AND THIN CALORIES

Calories from fat are more fattening than calories from protein or carbohydrates. Why is this so?

Fat contains a whopping 9 calories per gram, while carbohydrates and protein contain only 4 calories per gram, so that gram for gram fat is more than twice as fattening as carbohydrates or protein.

This is probably not news to you. Most people already know that an 8-ounce dish of ice cream has more calories than an 8-ounce dish of strawberries. It is what I am about to tell you about fat, however, that is news to a lot of people, since it is only recently that scientists have established this truth beyond a shadow of a doubt.

Fat is so easily digested by the human body, that almost no energy or calories are used up in digesting it. Only about 3 percent of the fat calories we consume are burned up during digestion. When we ingest carbohydrates or protein, on the other hand, about 20 percent of the calories they contain are used up in the digestion process.

What does all of this mean? Those of us who love fatty foods long thought that we could get away with eating them as long as we kept our calories down to a certain level. For example, if it took 1,800 calories to maintain Mary's weight, Mary assumed that she could consume her 1,800 calories any way she pleased. She could eat half of them in high-fat foods such as ice cream, fried foods, and red meat, and the other half in more nutritious low-fat foods. She falsely believed that it was the same thing as if she consumed most of her 1,800 calories in protein and carbohydrates.

The fact is, if Mary consumed half of her 1,800 calories in fat, she would end up digesting 180 calories more than if she consumed them in carbohydrates and protein. In a matter of three weeks, unless Mary burned up these extra calories by doing additional exercise, she would gain a pound of fat. (It only takes 3,000 excess calories to put on one pound of stored fat.) So you can see clearly that fat is the least desirable of food sources.

WE DO NEED SOME FAT IN OUR DIETS

Fat is not all bad. Insufficient body fat causes many problems. It is fat that forms cell membranes and surrounds our internal organs, protecting them from injury. Fat helps to insulate the body, keeping it warm on cold days. It is fat that comprises sex and natural steroid hormones. Without sufficient body fat, we would not be able to absorb and make use of calcium or vitamins D, E, A, and K.

But don't worry. It is almost impossible to suffer from fat deficiency if you live in America—or in any industrialized nation, for that matter—because most foods contain some fat. Even low-fat protein foods such as flounder, filet or skinless chicken breast have a certain amount of fat. (Eight ounces of flounder have 2 grams of fat; 8 ounces of chicken have 9 grams.) Even vegetable protein such as soybeans has a certain amount of fat. (Eight ounces of cooked soybeans have 10 grams.) It may surprise you to know that even fruit contains some fat. (An apple and a pear each have 1 gram.)

You can clearly see then that even if you vigilantly watched your diet, it would be impossible for you to eliminate all fat.

WHAT ABOUT CHOLESTEROL?

Cholesterol is fat in a waxlike form. It comes primarily in animal fats that are "saturated" or solid—for example, lard, butter, cheese, egg yolks, and the fat in meats.

Cholesterol is not all bad. It forms a major part of cell membranes, comprises the lining of the nerves, and composes much of the brain tissue. Clearly, a certain amount of cholesterol is necessary for good health. It becomes a problem, however, when it begins to line the arteries and blocks the flow of blood to the heart.

Most doctors agree that your cholesterol level should not exceed 200 milligrams. To further complicate the matter, there is "good cholesterol" and "bad cholesterol."

"Good cholesterol," high-density lipoprotein (HDL), functions *to remove* the cholesterol that can clog the arteries from the body and to transport it back to the liver for conversion into bile acids and subsequent elimination through the intestine.

"Bad cholesterol," low-density lipoprotein (LDL), is the cholesterol that can line the arterial walls, narrowing them and hindering the passage of blood to the organs of the body. It is easy to see how heart disease can develop from such a condition.

The dietary goal is to keep the LDL cholesterol level down to the point where it will not build up in the arteries, and to raise the HDL in order to keep LDL away from tissues and arteries.

Getting a True Cholesterol Count

When you get a cholesterol measurement, unless you ask for a breakdown, chances are you are given a single total. It may or may not be bad if that number is high, depending upon the breakdown. If the HDL is high, there may be no problem. However, if it is your LDL that is high, you could be in trouble.

In order to find out if you are at risk, ask your doctor for a "fractionated" cholesterol test. This test compares your HDL level to your total cholesterol count and gives you an index. The lower your index, the lower your risk. (An index of 4 or lower is considered low risk.) For example, if your total cholesterol level is 200 but your HDL is 50, your index is 4 (50 goes into 200 four times. If, on the other hand, your total cholesterol level is 200 but your HDL level is only 25, you are at greater risk—your risk index is 8 (25 goes into 200 eight times).

How to Raise Your HDL and Lower Your LDL

Scientists are now studying ways to raise the HDL level. At the present time, the only proven way to do this is to engage in weight training and aerobic activities, such as the ones described in this and other workout books.

To lower your LDL, eliminate all full-fat dairy products from your diet. Avoid all saturated fats, such as those found in butter, beef, veal, pork, lamb, and the skin of poultry. People with seriously high cholesterol levels are also advised to limit their intake of refined sugars and caffeine and to quit smoking.

What About Eggs?

If you enjoy eating eggs, there's good news. The American Heart Association recently reevaluated the cholesterol count in eggs and discovered that one egg contains only 213 milligrams of cholesterol, not 274, as previously reported. In effect, the new figures allow people who have to watch their cholesterol to have an additional egg per week. The former limit was three eggs per week. Now it is four eggs per week.

It is the egg yolk, not the white, that contains cholesterol. You can eat as many egg whites a week as you please. They are low in calories and are an excellent source of protein. Many people use one egg yolk and two or three egg whites in making scrambled or poached eggs.

PROTEIN: THE BASIC BODY-BUILDING MATERIAL

Protein is responsible for building and maintaining our basic body tissue. The muscles, internal organs, blood, hair, and nails are composed mainly of protein. In addition, protein regulates the water balance of the body.

Protein is made up of amino acids. There are twenty-two amino acids. Eight are produced naturally by the body. But to obtain the other fourteen, we must eat foods that contain them. Foods that can provide all of what are termed the essential amino acids (those the body cannot produce) are: egg whites, fish, poultry, milk and milk products, and red meat (in order of increasing fat content).

Vegetarians must combine foods to ensure satisfying their protein needs, as no single vegetable source provides all the essential amino acids. Rice and beans are the most common combination source of "complete" protein for vegetarians.

Since protein is best digested in small portions, it's better to eat a little at each meal rather than a lot all at once—20 to 30 grams at most. Try to eat protein two or three times a day.

CARBOHYDRATES: ENERGY FOOD

The human body depends primarily upon carbohydrates for energy. One of the first things you'll notice if you ever go on one of those high-protein, low-carbohydrate diets is that soon you feel weak. In addition. carbohydrates help to hold the proper balance of water in your muscles. People who go on high-protein. low-carbohydrate diets lose a lot of weight in the beginning stages of the diet because the muscles are forced to give up needed water. As a result. the scale shows a severe drop in weight (as much as ten pounds in one week). But the dieter quickly regains the water weight once normal eating is resumed.

Carbohydrates are also vital to proper brain functioning. In short. when your body is severely lacking in carbohydrates. you can't even think straight. You become nervous and irritable. Many a relationship has broken up and many a traffic accident has taken place because of a low-carbohydrate diet.

When carbohydrates are consumed. they are immediately broken down by the digestive system into glucose. or what is commonly called "blood sugar." It is glucose that supplies your central nervous system with energy.

There are two types of carbohydrates: simple and complex. Simple carbohydrates (sugars) are found in natural foods such as fruit and in processed foods such as jams. jellies. candies. and white flour.

Simple Carbohydrates

For years it was thought that there was a great deal of difference in the way the body reacts to processed simple carbohydrates such as refined sugar and natural simple carbohydrates such as fruit. For example, it was believed that if you ate a teaspoon of sugar in a candy bar, your blood sugar would immediately rise. You would experience a sudden burst of energy then, later on, a drop in energy. But if you ate a piece of fruit such as a banana you would experience no corresponding energy boost and drop.

Sugar is not as bad as we thought it was. Recent research has shown that you get the same energy boost. whether you consume a simple carbohydrate sugar or fruit. And as long as you don't eat these foods on an empty stomach, you won't get a severe energy drop. In addition, researchers have not been able to come up with any proof whatsoever that sugar is addictive. In fact, not one study has been able to demonstrate scientifically that you experience withdrawal symptoms when you stop consuming sugar.

The facts are clear. Whether you consume refined sugar or natural sugar in fruit, the results are the same. The sugar is converted into glucose and used as an immediate source of energy. The sugar in fruit (fructose, sucrose, and glucose) and the sugar in most candies are almost identical. They are both simple sugar molecules and are quickly digested.

If this is true, is it okay to stop eating fruit and eat sweets instead, as long as they are low in fat? Of course not. Fruits contain lots of nutrients (vitamins, minerals, and fiber) not found in processed sweets. On the other hand, you need not totally eliminate sweets from your diet. In fact, it's a good idea to treat yourself to a sweet once in a while. A sweet, low-fat treat such as jam, jelly, or hard candy can help you feel a little less deprived if you have really been watching your fat. A teaspoon of regular jam or jelly contains only about 18 calories, with virtually no fat. Sometimes such a treat may be just the thing to prevent you from indulging in a high-fat treat such as ice cream or doughnuts.

The Superiority of Complex Carbohydrates

Complex carbohydrates, in the form of grains and vegetables, are preferable to simple carbohydrates because they consist of multiple natural sugar molecules. It takes the digestive system more time to break them down than it does to break down simple carbohydrate molecules. As a result, instead of delivering a quick energy burst, these carbohydrates dole out a slowly released, continuing supply of energy.

FIBER

There are two kinds of fiber—soluble and insoluble.

Many carbohydrates have a high soluble fiber content. The body can digest soluble fiber, which is found in foods such as oat bran, psyllium, beans, vegetables, and fruits. Some studies have shown that daily ingestion of as little as 6 grams of this type of fiber helps to lower cholesterol and blood sugar levels.

The body cannot digest insoluble fiber such as whole wheat and wheat bran. But insoluble fiber is instrumental in the prevention of constipation, diverticulosis, and colon cancer.

Here's how it works: Insoluble fiber helps to enlarge and loosen the stool, facilitating easy passage. Because the stool is not forced to remain a long time in the intestinal track, undue irritation of the intestinal wall is prevented, and diverticulosis (a condition in which small bulges develop in the lining of the large intestine) is avoided. Because the fiber also helps to dilute toxic agents in the bowel, colon cancer is less likely.

The Calorie Bonus in Fiber

When you consume a high-fiber product, you can automatically deduct about 20 percent of the calories, because cellulose, a main compound of insoluble fiber, cannot be digested by the human body.

When the calories for a given complex carbohydrate are calculated, the calories of the cellulose content of that food are included in the calculation. But since the body is not capable of digesting cellulose (our intestines lack the enzymes required to break down this substance), these calories cannot be absorbed or used by the body. If you are consuming a high-fiber food, you can generally count on getting a 20 percent calorie bonus.

VITAMINS AND MINERALS

If you eat a generous supply of the fruits and vegetables, fish, chicken, and low-fat dairy products suggested in this chapter, you will suffer no vitamin or mineral deficiency and will not need to take supplements. (Of course, you should follow your doctor's advice on this subject.)

I do not use vitamins or food supplements. I have always felt that taking vitamins confuses the body's natural survival system, making it less likely to crave the natural foods containing needed vitamins and minerals. Medical authorities agree. It is always better to get your nutrients through your food rather than in concentrated extracts.

All I can do is offer you my personal experience and let you make your own decision. I am well into my forties and about as healthy as a human being can be. Not everyone is the same, and we all have different health histories, so please go by your particular needs. Do not feel obligated to follow in my footsteps.

We all need a balanced diet of vitamins—A, B-complex (B_1, B_2, B_6, B_{12}, niacin), C, D, and E. These organic substances are found for the most part in yellow and green leafy vegetables, rice, whole grains, fish, poultry, and beef. We also need a generous supply of minerals, including iron, magnesium, phosphorus, potassium, sodium, and calcium. These nutrients are found in foods such as whole grains, green vegetables, fruit, fish, poultry, organ meats, and beef.

Calcium

The mineral calcium is largely responsible for keeping our bones strong and healthy. A calcium deficiency can cause brittle, easily broken bones, especially after age thirty.

You may want to take a calcium supplement just to be on the safe side. Most doctors recommend a 1,500-milligram tablet daily, although the United States government suggests only between 800 and 1,200 milligrams daily.

I do not take calcium supplements. Instead I do the weight-bearing exercises discussed in this book and eat high-calcium foods. It has been demonstrated that weight-bearing exercises help to strengthen and thicken bones.

To make sure you eat a high-calcium diet, include a generous amount of the foods suggested among the "unlimited" carbohydrates, the proteins, or the starchy carbohydrates recommended in the Fat-Burning Eating Plan outlined in this chapter.

The following foods contain 100 milligrams of calcium:

1 cup broccoli	⅔ cup wheat cereal
1 cup kale	1 cup farina
1 cup collard greens	1 cup skim milk
1 cup turnip greens	⅔ cup low-fat cottage cheese
10 okra pods	8 ounces plain low-fat yogurt
⅔ cup oatmeal	1 cup cooked soybeans

If you select foods from the above list every day, you should have no trouble consuming your daily requirement of calcium.

Sodium

The mineral sodium is vital to our physical well-being. Together with potassium, it helps to regulate body fluids and maintain the acid-alkali balance of the blood, as well as helps the muscles contract.

Although there is no official recommended amount of sodium, a generally acceptable range is between 1,500 and 2,500 milligrams daily.

A deficiency in sodium can result in muscle cramping, intestinal gas, nausea, and muscle shrinkage. Too much sodium in the diet, on the other hand, can result in water retention (sodium holds up to fifty times its own weight in water) and high blood pressure.

It is almost impossible to suffer from sodium deficiency unless you are also suffering from malnutrition, because nearly everything we eat contains some sodium. For example, there are 59 milligrams of sodium in an 8-ounce glass of club soda, 2.5 milligrams in a cup of coffee, 10 milligrams in a glass of tap water, 121 milligrams in a slice of whole wheat bread, 150 milligrams in an 8-ounce chicken breast, 16 milligrams in a cup of cooked broccoli, 6 milligrams in a boiled potato, 16 milligrams in a cup of brown rice, and 1 milligram in an orange.

Many foods contain an excessive amount of sodium. Canned soups contain about 1,000 milligrams per cup. Frozen dinners, even "diet" dinners, usually contain about 1,000 milligrams per serving. Condiments, such as ketchup, mustard, and Worcestershire sauce are notoriously high in sodium (500 to

1,000 milligrams per tablespoon), as are Chinese foods, smoked foods, and pizza (approximately 1,000 milligrams per 8-ounce serving).

Sodium and Water Retention

If you follow the suggested Fat-Burning Eating Plan, chances are you will not be in danger of consuming too much sodium. But what if you wish to indulge yourself and eat high-sodium, low-calorie foods such as frozen diet dinners, canned soups, pickles, Chinese foods, and so on? With your doctor's permission, you may, unless, of course, you have high blood pressure. You will not gain permanent weight. You will temporarily gain a few pounds of water weight, but in a matter of days (probably five) you can get rid of it by cutting down on your sodium.

Until you lose the three to five pounds of water, you will look, feel, and weigh "fatter," but in reality, you will not be fatter. You will be heavier and bigger—but only until you eliminate the water. If you don't mind looking or feeling a little fatter once in a while, and if you don't let it discourage you from your diet (that is, you don't weigh yourself and say, "Oh my goodness, I gained two pounds. I might as well go out and eat a quart of ice cream"), then feel free to indulge in high-sodium, low-fat foods once in a while. It may provide you with needed relief from discipline. At least you know that it will take only five days to get rid of those three pounds of water, instead of the five weeks it might take you to get rid of the three pounds of fat you would put on if you indulged in high-fat foods instead.

WATER

Water is the major transporter of nutrients throughout the body. We need water for absorption, digestion, circulation, excretion, and the elimination of wastes. Two-thirds of our body weight consists of water.

The more water you drink, the less you will retain, because water helps to neutralize the sodium in your system. As a matter of fact, when doctors prescribe a daily allowance of sodium, they usually base their decision upon how much water the individual regularly consumes.

Drinking water is equivalent to giving the internal organs a shower. How sad that some people shower their inner bodies only with coffee, cola, or colored diet sodas! Try to drink five 8-ounce glasses of water daily—one upon rising, one before each meal, and one before bedtime.

Drinking water in this manner will help to decrease your appetite, too. Many times when we think we're hungry, we're really not. We're actually thirsty. Here's how it works.

If you haven't been drinking enough water, your body becomes slightly dehydrated. When this happens, if you don't think of giving it water, your body will lead you to food, because most foods contain some water.

What kind of water should you drink? Tap water is fine, although some say it is dangerously polluted. I drink it without worry, although sometimes I drink bottled water just for a change. I don't like water, and drinking bottled water helps me to think I am not drinking water. It seems special if it's in the bottle. It also seems to taste better.

If you are concerned with the pollutants found in tap water, you can get a home purification system or rely on bottled water, but by all means, drink your water!

HOW TO MAKE SURE YOU GET ENOUGH FIBER AND NUTRIENTS IN YOUR DIET

Follow the eating guidelines set forth in the following paragraphs, and you will get more than your minimum daily requirement of all the vitamins and minerals and fiber you need. Your new way of eating is going to be to "pig out" on a large bowl of delicious steamed or cold vegetables or on a large, luscious salad.

You will have no trouble getting your daily requirement of nutrients and, what's more, you won't have to be self-conscious about it. You can eat and enjoy your life without having to calculate everything. The only food element you will have to calculate and vigilantly watch is fat.

GETTING DOWN TO BUSINESS

From this moment on, I want you to be on the alert to fats in your diet. Most food labels indicate fat content in grams rather than in calories. If a food is not labeled, look up its fat content in *The Nutrition Almanac* (see bibliography).

You are allowed to have no more than 20 to 30 grams of fat per day if you want to burn the excess fat from your body. You must never put anything in your mouth without knowing how many grams of fat are contained in that food. After a few weeks, you won't have to check too often, because you will have learned that certain foods (fruits and vegetables) contain virtually no fat.

You'll also quickly realize that butter, oil, mayonnaise, full-fat dairy products, all cheeses, red meats, chocolate, doughnuts, and most cakes and pies are out of the question. Eliminate fried foods as well. Just one tablespoon of cooking oil has 14 grams of fat. That's almost half your maximum daily fat allowance. You could bake or broil the food instead and save your fat allotment for other things.

If you choose water-packed tuna instead of tuna in oil, you save 7 grams of fat on every 3 ½-ounce portion. If you choose skim milk over regular milk, you save 3 grams of fat for every 8-ounce glass you consume. Since cheeses in general are so high in fat, I advise you to avoid them altogether, except for low-fat cottage cheese.

An 8-ounce fast food hamburger has a grand total of 23 grams of fat. If you choose broiled fish instead, you will be consuming only about 3 grams of fat. See how easy it is to limit fat from your diet once you become "fat aware"?

Surprisingly, many frozen dinners have as much as 25 grams of fat. Read the labels. The information is there. You will be amazed to see that even so-called "diet" dinners are guilty of this offense.

For your information, here is a list of high-fat foods. Except for the foods marked with an asterisk, included for contrast, completely eliminate these foods from your diet until you have reached your weight goal. Then, as I'll explain later, you can indulge in any or all of them *once a week*.

GRAMS FAT

1 cup rich ice cream	24
1 ounce American cheese	9
1 ounce Swiss cheese	8
1 ounce cheddar cheese	9
1 ounce part-skim mozzarella	5
8 ounces regular milk	8
8 ounces 2% fat milk	5
*8 ounces 1% fat milk	2.5
*8 ounces skim milk	1
1 chocolate chip cookie	3
1 doughnut	27
2 ounces potato chips	20
½ cup peanuts	36
6 ounces cooked spareribs	51
6 ounces cooked loin of lamb	16
6 ounces sausage	62

Again, you can find out the fat content of almost any food by reading the label or looking it up in *The Nutrition Almanac* (see bibliography).

THE FAT-BURNING EATING PLAN: BASIC GUIDELINES

I deliberately call this the Fat-Burning Eating Plan rather than the Fat-Burning Diet because the word *diet* has come to have negative connotations. Most of us associate the word *diet* with deprivation, and rightly so. Chances are you have embarked upon at least one diet that caused you to starve yourself day after day with little permanent reward.

The word *diet* means "one's customary, prescribed food." Since the starvation "diets" one goes on by no means consist of customary food, I think they are more properly called "deprivations," not diets.

The Fat-Burning Eating Plan, on the other hand, is a diet in the truest sense of the word. It is in fact a normal, happy, healthy way of eating that will quickly become natural to you. However, just because most people do get negative flashbacks when the word *diet* is mentioned, I shall call this new fat-burning food program an eating plan and not a diet.

The following twelve guidelines are all you need to know in order to follow the Fat-Burning Eating Plan. Make yourself a photocopy of them, and carry them with you. Read them daily until you have the information fixed in your mind.

1. Do not consume more than 30 grams of fat a day. If possible, while trying to lose weight, keep your fat intake closer to 20 grams a day. Avoid any food that is more than 25 percent fat. Read labels and check *The Nutrition Almanac* for the fat content of foods. The following foods contain between 50 percent and 100 percent fat: all hard cheeses; full-fat cottage cheese, milk, and milk products; ice cream; butter; mayonnaise; oils; red meats such as beef, pork, lamb; sausage; the skin of poultry; avocados; nuts; potato chips; chocolate. There are many others. Never put anything in your mouth without checking first.

2. Never deny yourself food when you are hungry. Carry snack foods with you in plastic containers or food storage bags. You can snack freely on "unlimited" complex carbohydrates like bamboo shoots, broccoli, brussels sprouts, cabbage, carrots, cauliflower, celery, chard, cucumber, eggplant, green beans, kale, lettuce (any kind), mushrooms, mustard greens, onions, peppers (all colors), radishes, spinach, squash (all kinds), tomatoes, turnips, watercress, and zucchini.

3. As a general rule, eat starchy complex carbohydrates only twice a day: one bagel, two slices of bread, one bran or corn muffin, one cup of any cereal, two cups of puffed wheat or puffed rice, one cup of pasta, one cup of white

or brown rice, one large potato, one cup of corn, peas or beets. Starchy carbohydrates tend to satisfy hunger. They also have a calming effect, but they slow the metabolism slightly. Save the starchy complex carbohydrates for when you are very hungry or when you want to relax.

4. If you are extremely hungry, rather than choose a high-fat food, select a third or even fourth starchy complex carbohydrate. The calorie count is much lower, and you will not slow down your metabolism nearly as much as you will if you eat a fatty food. Substitute a starchy complex carbohydrate for 10 grams of your fat allotment. That is, if you consume 20 grams of fat and are still hungry, rather than take advantage of the 10 additional allowed fat grams, it's better to have another starchy carbohydrate.

5. Eat protein at least twice a day. Good sources of low-fat protein are egg whites, white-meat chicken or turkey, low-fat cottage cheese, low-fat or nonfat yogurt, and fish. Choose low-fat fish like abalone, bass, clams, cod, flounder, halibut, perch, pike, pollock, snapper, and tuna in water. Avoid fatty fish such as bluefish, carp, catfish, herring, mackerel, salmon, shad, swordfish, trout, and whitefish. If you are concerned with cholesterol, avoid low-fat, but high-cholesterol, sea food such as crab, lobster, and shrimp.

6. Eat at least five times a day. Have three full meals and two snacks. Try not to go without eating for more than four hours. This will prevent overeating at your next meal and keep your metabolism high.

7. You may have two to four fruits per day. For a quick energy boost, eat a piece of fruit, but never on an empty stomach. (Eating a simple carbohydrate on an empty stomach may give you a quick energy burst, but it will be followed by a letdown twenty minutes later. Instead, on an empty stomach eat complex carbohydrates or protein.) Use fruit to satisfy a craving for sweets. You may occasionally substitute a teaspoon of jam or jelly or your favorite low-fat hard candy for the fruit. Don't use processed sugar or a product high in processed sugar more than once every other day. Fruit has vitamins, minerals, and fiber that processed sugar does not provide.

8. Drink five 8-ounce glasses of water a day. The best plan is to drink a glass upon rising, a glass with every meal, and a glass just before bedtime.

9. Never eat anything that is fried. You must broil, boil, steam, or poach everything, and never in butter, oil, or any other fatty substance.

10. Don't starve yourself. Never consume less than 1,000 calories a day. That

will slow down your metabolism and you will have deprived yourself for nothing because you will lose less weight than you would have if you had kept your calories up to between 1,250 and 1,800. You need not count calories on this diet, but if you are constantly hungry, add them up just to make sure you are not going below 1,000.

11. Take a ten-minute walk after at least one of your three meals, preferably after all three.

12. Be alert to your intake of sodium. Sodium causes water retention. Although the resulting weight gain is not permanent, when you retain water you feel fat and that feeling can discourage you if you're trying to lose weight. On the other hand, assuming you do not suffer from high blood pressure, a high-sodium, low-fat treat such as a pickle, canned soup, or Chinese food may provide a welcome relief from ordinary foods. This relief may help you to avoid eating high-fat foods.

WHY YOU WILL LOSE WEIGHT IF YOU FOLLOW THIS EATING PLAN

1. Experts believe that it is virtually impossible to get or be fat if you do not eat fat.

2. If you are keeping your fat intake low (no more than 30 grams of fat per day) you will automatically be cutting down your calories, too! Whether we realize it or not, most of the "naughty" foods we like to eat are comprised of high-calorie fats.

3. Although you are allowed to eat as much as you please of certain complex carbohydrates, you will not be consuming enough calories to store up fat, for two reasons: These "unlimited" complex carbohydrates are all low-calorie foods, and a person can eat just so much of one thing without getting tired of it. You will automatically limit yourself after a while.

4. Fat slows down your metabolism. Since you will be limiting your fat, your metabolism will speed up and you will be burning more calories twenty-four hours a day.

5. Since you've cut down on your fat intake so drastically, you will be consuming fewer calories than you need to use during the course of a day. Your body will begin to use its stored fat for energy.

HOW FAST WILL YOU LOSE WEIGHT?

The more overweight you are, the faster you will lose the weight. Why is this the case? The heavier you are, the greater the calorie deficit you will be creating. In other words, if you are fifty pounds overweight and you begin to follow the Fat-Burning Eating Plan, you will be consuming between 1,250 and 1,800 calories. A person who is only ten pounds overweight will be consuming the same 1,250 to 1,800 calories. The heavier person will lose more, because it takes more calories to sustain a heavier weight (the deficit is greater).

If you are very much overweight, you can count on losing an average of a pound and a half to two pounds a week. If you are between one and fifteen pounds overweight, you will lose an average of a half a pound to a pound and a half a week, over a period of about twelve weeks. This is a conservative estimate. You may even lose faster.

HOW MUCH FAT DO YOU CONSUME ON A DAILY BASIS?

Be honest. How many grams of fat do you consume on a daily basis now, when you are not making a special effort to watch what you eat? Write down every single thing you ate yesterday, including the milk in your coffee—everything. Now add up the grams of fat contained in each food item (consult *The Nutrition Almanac*).

I'll bet you consumed at least 50 grams of fat—probably more. Maybe you skipped breakfast, then had a Burger King hamburger (13 grams of fat) and french fries (11 grams of fat) with a vanilla shake (11 grams of fat) for lunch. For dinner, you may have had one roasted chicken breast with skin (8 grams of fat) and 2 tablespoons of Italian salad dressing on your salad (15 grams of fat). Later in the evening, you had a cup of chocolate ice cream (15 grams of fat). So far, we have a grand total of 76 grams of fat. You have consumed more than double the amount allowed on the Fat-Burning Eating Plan.

Anyone knows that beef and ice cream are high-fat foods. But you can easily consume more than the proper amount of fat even if you avoid these obvious fat culprits. All you have to do is have a bagel and cream cheese for breakfast, a cup of regular cottage cheese with coffee and regular milk for lunch, and fried flounder and broccoli au gratin (with cheese) for dinner. You will have consumed almost 50 grams of fat, twenty more than your maximum allowance.

A young lady who was following the Fat-Burning Workout was having a problem losing her last seven pounds. As it turned out, she was making some mistakes. First, she used full-fat milk in her coffee, and she drank plenty of coffee and liked it light. Next, she put two to three tablespoons of oil or regular salad dressing on her salad. Next, she ate full-fat cottage cheese for lunch every day, because the restaurant near her place of business didn't carry the low-fat variation, and she didn't think it would matter much if she ignored that one rule. Let's look why even a few small mistakes can stop you from losing the body fat you want to lose.

There are 8 grams of fat in a cup of full-fat milk, whereas there is only 1 gram of fat in a cup of skim milk. There are 42 grams of fat in three tablespoons of oil, whereas there is no fat in vinegar, lemon juice, and spices. There are 10 grams of fat in a cup of regular cottage cheese, whereas there are only 2 grams of fat in low-fat cottage cheese. In total, she was consuming 56 unnecessary grams of fat. Notice that we did not even calculate her breakfast or dinner, which must contain some fat, even if she was sticking to the Fat-Burning Eating Plan for these meals, as she says she was.

Fifty-eight grams of additional fat will certainly sabotage your fat-loss plan. That's 522 of the fattest calories possible, and they will cling to your hips, buttocks, thighs, and abdominal area. So don't fool around with fat. Be a fat detective. That's the only way this eating plan will work to rid you of your excess body fat.

DAILY MEAL PLANS

Every day, you will eat three main meals and two snacks. Remember: You will have at least two protein portions a day, and you will have only two starchy carbohydrates. You will have no more than 20 to 30 grams of fat a day. And don't forget your glass of water before each meal.

Note: Recent studies indicate that one should consume a minimum of two and a half cups of vegetables daily in order to improve health, decrease chances of getting cancer, and slow down the aging process.

Sample Meal Plan # 1

Breakfast

1 egg yolk and 2 or 3 egg whites poached, scrambled, or soft or hard boiled.
6 ounces grapefruit or orange juice

Snack

1 fruit
unlimited complex carbohydrates (vegetables)

Lunch

6 ounces water-packed tuna salad (mix tuna with onion, cucumber, red pepper,
    vinegar, and black pepper) on 2 slices of whole wheat toast
large tossed salad (unlimited complex carbohydrates) with no oil dressing
coffee, tea, or no-calorie soda

Snack

unlimited complex carbohydrates
1 fruit

Dinner

8 ounces broiled skinless chicken breast
2 cups assorted unlimited complex carbohydrates
large tossed salad
½ grapefruit
no-calorie beverage

Snack

1 slice whole wheat toast
1 tablespoon jelly
6-ounce glass tomato juice (low-sodium if you care)

Sample Meal Plan # 2

Breakfast

1 bran muffin and 1 teaspoon of jelly
1 orange
coffee or tea or no-calorie beverage

Snack

1 8-ounce container low-fat yogurt

Lunch

1 cup low-fat cottage cheese on a bed of lettuce
unsweetened fruit salad
coffee or tea or no-calorie beverage

Dinner

8 ounces broiled flounder
1 cup spaghetti and 4 ounces tomato sauce
2 cups unlimited complex carbohydrates
large tossed salad
no-calorie beverage

Snack

unlimited complex carbohydrates

Sample Meal Plan # 3

Breakfast

1 cup shredded wheat cereal
1 cup skim milk
8 ounces strawberries
no-calorie beverage

Snack

unlimited complex carbohydrates

Lunch

6 ounces chicken chunks
large tossed salad
unlimited complex carbohydrates
no-calorie beverage

Dinner

8 ounces broiled halibut
1 baked potato and 2 tablespoons plain yogurt
2 cups unlimited complex carbohydrates
large tossed salad
unsweetened gelatin
no-calorie beverage

Snack

1 cup cherries
unlimited complex carbohydrates

Guess what? Each of the above meals contains only half of your allowed fat grams. This leaves you with 15 grams of fat to fool around with. You can indulge in one of the following each day if you wish:

1 tablespoon vegetable oil on the salad—14 grams of fat
1 tablespoon regular Italian salad dressing—7 grams of fat
1 tablespoon cream cheese on the bagel—10 grams of fat
1 tablespoon butter on the toast—12.3 grams of fat
1 tablespoon mayonnaise on the tuna salad—11 grams of fat
1 tablespoon sour cream on the potato—2.5 grams of fat

Even though you'll be within your fat allowance when adding some of these items, it would be better to forgo the fat and simply consume more unlimited complex carbohydrates. Your next best bet is to consume another portion of starchy carbohydrates. Remember, the less fat you eat, the faster you will burn the fat off your body, because your body will use up its fat stores for necessary energy.

Although I have laid out a plan specifying three meals and two snacks, you may feel free to have additional snacks of unlimited complex carbohydrates any time you are hungry.

THE FAT-BURNING MAINTENANCE PLAN

Once you have reached your goal, continue to eat the same way, only now you may have a starchy carbohydrate three times a day, and you may up your fat consumption to 30 to 35 grams a day. In addition, you may eat whatever you wish one day a week.

In order to make sure that you don't gain back the fat, if you indulge in high-fat foods on your one free eating day, do some additional exercise to burn off the fat the next day, or the day after at the latest. For example, if you consumed 54 grams of fat instead of your allotted 30 to 35 grams of fat, you can run for twenty minutes. You will burn off 24 grams of fat, or 216 calories. (Running for twenty minutes burns approximately 220 calories.) See chapter 9 for additional fat-burning aerobic exercises.

VACATIONS

When you go on vacation, you have some choices. You can maintain your low-fat eating plan while away if you choose. There's no reason not to. These days, with a high health consciousness in most resorts and restaurants, it isn't difficult to get low-fat foods. You can order broiled fish or chicken, steamed vegetables, a baked potato, pasta or rice, a tossed salad, and so on. Just be sure to request that the food is cooked and served with no butter or oil.

If you feel like indulging a little, eat whatever you please every other day, up to fourteen days. This will mean that you have indulged in high-fat foods on seven different days. In order to get back on track after your vacation, you'll have to sacrifice a few weeks of free eating days—about three or four.

When you return home, resume the regular Fat Burning Eating Plan until you feel that you have gotten rid of any excess fat. If you want to speed up your progress, you can always do some of the aerobic exercises described in chapter 9.

It isn't a good idea to stop working out for more than one week. If you're going to be away for longer than that, why not do the 12-Minute Total-Body Workout? (See bibliography.) All you have to do is carry your three-pound dumbbells with you. I do it all the time. In fact, since that workout is so convenient and quick, I never stop working out totally. Even if I go away for three days, I take my three-pound dumbbells. It makes me feel alert and alive, and I feel fit and energetic all day long.

If you stop working out completely, you will feel as if something is missing. You won't have that natural high. Your body will feel slightly sluggish. Why give up that natural high when all you have to do is invest twelve minutes a day to feel your best?

THE MOMENT YOU FEEL THAT YOU ARE REGAINING THE FAT

If you have been using the Fat-Burning Workout, but notice that you're gaining weight—maybe your clothing is getting tighter—face the facts. It's time to take action before things get worse.

Don't wait until the situation gets out of hand. Immediately return to the regular Fat-Burning Eating Plan, and if you're not already doing it, step up your Fat-Burning Workout to the Intensity or Insanity plan. If you're ambitious, you may even want to add in some of the additional fat-burning aerobic exercises discussed in chapter 9.

Once you reach your ideal fat and fitness level, don't be afraid to return to the maintenance plan. If you try to maintain a rigid low-fat diet all year round, you may find yourself unconsciously putting fatty foods in your mouth while you're daydreaming (perhaps while standing at the refrigerator or while cooking dinner). It's much better to give your body occasional breaks from a very strict eating plan. Why is this so?

The human body and mind like variation. If you try to turn yourself into a robot, your body and mind will find a way to sabotage you just to experience change. In addition, if you remain on a strict eating plan and work out all year round, there will be no place to go when you want to crack down on yourself. You will have already been doing everything you possibly can.

LOW-FAT EATING ON THE RUN

Carry unlimited complex carbohydrates with you in a baggy or a plastic container. Stop at a fruit and vegetable stand to purchase red peppers, cucumbers, apples, pears, peaches, strawberries, or other fruit or vegetable. Stop at a grocery store and purchase yogurt, cottage cheese, raisins, pretzels, juice, a white-meat chicken or turkey sandwich on whole wheat toast, or some other low-fat food.

If you live in a big city and are rushing from one appointment to the next and have no time for lunch, you may purchase one of those luscious soft pretzels and a diet soda, or have a bagel with no butter. These are legitimate starchy carbohydrates, and they will prevent you from feeling starved and becoming irritable at your next appointment. They will also stop you from overeating at your next meal, and will help to prevent your metabolism from slowing down.

You may think it strange to have to use discipline to eat when you're not even thinking of food, but do it. If you don't, you'll slow down your progress. This is very important.

If you order lunch in, use the guidelines discussed below.

LOW-FAT DINING OUT

No problem. Order whatever you want broiled, baked, boiled, or poached without butter, cream, or oil of any kind. Order pasta with tomato sauce, baked potatoes, fish, chicken, vegetables, salads. Watch the soups. You really have no way of telling how much fat is contained in them unless you see the fat content on a can, and most restaurants don't use canned soups. They are also high in sodium.

Many restaurants have low-calorie meals, but be careful. Even though the calories may be low, the fat grams may be high. Ask if the restaurant has a fat-gram count. If not, order according to what you already know about fats.

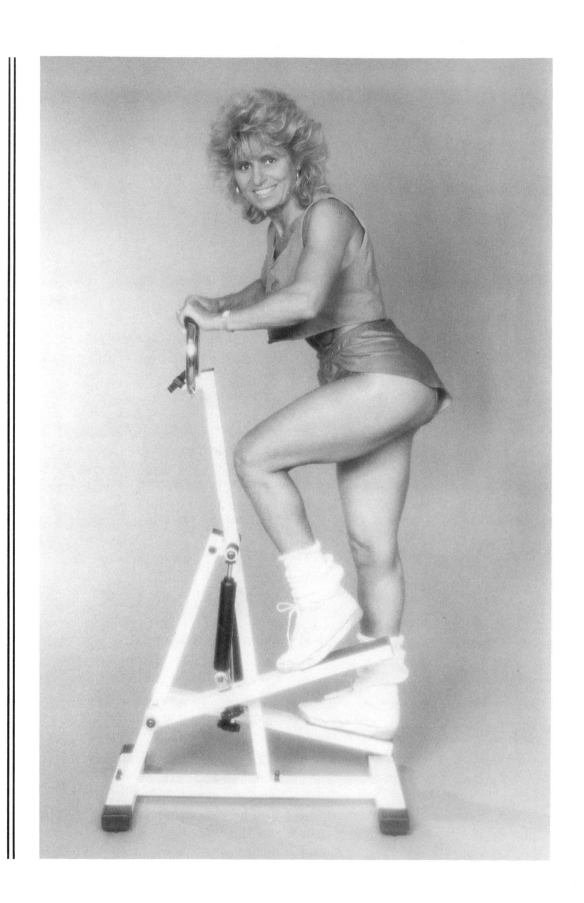

9 | WORKING OVERTIME

In this chapter you will find out how to accelerate the elimination of your excess body fat, how to increase your aerobic fitness, how to find ways to burn fat during the course of a typical busy work day, and how to speed up your progress in reshaping your troublesome body parts.

WHY BOTHER WITH THE EXTRAS?

Exercise speeds up your metabolism for up to two hours after you have worked out. You burn additional calories not only when you are exercising, but also after you stop exercising. As an added bonus, the increase in metabolism makes you feel more energetic, so that you are more inclined to move rather than stay still, stand rather than sit, and trot rather than drag your body along in a slow walk. This increase in energy will then also help you to burn additional calories, because the more you move, the more calories you burn.

In addition, exercise helps to decrease your appetite. It has been demonstrated that exercise helps to stabilize the insulin level in your blood, which helps to control your appetite.

So think of it this way: Every time you invest a little extra time in exercise, you get a multiple return for your effort. Your small investment quickly turns into a big fat-burning bargain.

AEROBIC ACTIVITIES

As noted earlier, the Fat-Burning Workout is itself an aerobic activity. As you know, it is also a body-shaping workout. It accomplishes two goals at once: It burns fat and it shapes the body. There are other activities that can be added to the Fat-Burning Workout that are not body-shaping activities, but strictly aerobic. You can use these activities to burn additional fat and to help condition your heart and lungs. In addition, these exercises will help to increase your stamina for the Fat-Burning Workout itself.

As discussed before, in order to be considered aerobic, an exercise must get your pulse rate up to between 70 and 85 percent of its capacity and keep it there for twenty minutes. However, many fitness experts now feel that a sustained pulse rate of 60 percent of maximum for even twelve minutes has a significant aerobic effect. So don't assume that unless you take a full twenty minutes or your heart is racing that it's a waste of time to exercise. (We'll talk more about this later in the chapter.)

In order to determine your minimum and maximum aerobic pulse rate, subtract your age from 220. Then multiply the result by 60 percent. This will give you the bare minimum aerobic effect. Now multiply the figure by 70 percent. This will be your traditional minimum for an aerobic effect. Now multiply the figure by 80 percent. This will put you in the high aerobic range. Now multiply it by 85 percent. This will bring you to your maximum aerobic capacity.

BREAKING IN GENTLY

In order to ensure that you won't overstress your heart and lungs, it is most important that you break in gently to aerobic activities. Here is a simple break-in schedule.

Week 1: three to five minutes
Week 2: five to seven minutes
Week 3: seven to ten minutes
Week 4: ten to fifteen minutes
Week 5: fifteen to twenty minutes
Week 6: twenty to twenty-five minutes
Week 7: twenty-five to thirty minutes

You should work from the lower end of the scale upward, so that by the end of the week you are at the higher end of the scale. For example, on the first day of week one, you may run (or jump rope or ride a bike or swim) for three minutes. On the next day, you may run for four minutes, and by the end of the week, you may run for five minutes. Then on week two, you may start with five minutes and work your way up to seven minutes by the end of the week, and so on.

Remember, there is no rush. Take your time and enjoy what you're doing. In the long run, it won't matter if it took you a little longer to build up to a twenty-minute run, jump, ride, or swim. But it can be detrimental if you try to rush it so that you hyperventilate and feel as if you are having a heart attack. Then you will want to quit the program.

It took you a long time to get out of shape, whether you realize it or not. You weren't aware of what was happening then because you were blissfully enjoying the lazy life. It will take you less time to get into shape than it did to get out of shape. But now you are self-conscious. Now you are working hard. Every minute seems an hour. Every week seems a month. Realize this and be patient with yourself. Be sensible. Give it time.

PICKING AN AEROBIC ACTIVITY

In selecting an aerobic activity, remember that convenience and enjoyment are the keys. For me, running or walking fast are both convenient and enjoyable, so they are my first choices. My second choices are jumping rope or riding the stationary bicycle. I also love to use the stair climbing machine and the Nordic Track machine.

Running

I've run outdoors all over the world, from Italy to Israel to Africa. I must admit, I got lost a few times, and that was really frightening especially when no one could give me directions that I could understand. Finally, I learned a simple survival trick. Since I don't have a great sense of direction, I look at my watch and run for ten minutes in one direction, then turn around and run back for ten minutes, and I'm right back where I started.

If the road ends before my ten minutes are up, rather than make a turn and risk getting lost, I look at my watch at that point and turn back. Then, when I get back to where I started, I either repeat the route or go in another direction for a given number of minutes.

But what happens when you just don't want to go out of doors and run, for

184

whatever reason? It may be zero degrees outside, and the streets may be glazed with ice. Or you may just not be in the mood to go out of doors. In this case, fortunately, there are other options.

Rope Jumping

To me, rope jumping is the most convenient aerobic activity in existence. All you need is an inexpensive, lightweight rope. Even a child's rope that can be purchased in any five and dime store will do. You can carry the rope with you anywhere in the world, and you can jump in the privacy of your room, out on a terrace or balcony, or in the back yard. You can do it to silence, to the sound of music, or while watching television.

I've jumped rope on the balcony of my room in many a Grand Hotel, on a hotel balcony on the French Riviera, on a terrace at Club Med, and in the back yards or bedrooms of friends I have stayed with. Why, I've even jumped rope on the decks of various ocean liners, rather than vault over people with the other runners who were busily going around in circles.

A variation of rope jumping is trampoline jumping. Trampolines made especially for this purpose are inexpensive and can be purchased in any sporting goods store. They are no more than two and a half feet in diameter and can easily be stored under a bed. Trampolines are especially convenient if you live in an apartment building and are concerned about disturbing your downstairs neighbors.

Bicycling

A very practical aerobic activity is riding the stationary bicycle. These days, a stationary bicycle can be purchased for a reasonable price. I like to ride the bicycle when I'm bored with running or jumping but still want to do some additional aerobic work because I've gone overboard and put on more fat than is comfortable for me. I can ride the bike and watch TV, or listen to music or informational tapes.

The advantage of a stationary bicycle over riding outdoors is convenience and consistency. You need not depend upon the weather, and you can ride any time, night or day, without fear or danger. You don't have to worry about being held back by traffic or pedestrians, so you can keep up your pace and ensure that you are getting the full fat-burning aerobic effect from your workout.

The Stair Machine

Another interesting aerobic option is the stair machine. Years ago, this machine was largely unavailable to the public for home use because of its expense. However, with the increasing popularity of home exercise equipment, many companies are now manufacturing models that are specially designed for home use, and are less expensive. In fact, if you really want to save money, you can buy a light-duty model that works for anyone under 160 pounds.

Of course, one need not use a machine to run stairs. It is perfectly acceptable to run up and down regular stairs instead. However, it is not always as convenient. Most of us do not have six flights of stairs in our home—and we would be too bored to run up and down the one flight we do have—so we would have to drive somewhere else to find them. Once there, we would have to put up with curious onlookers. So for the sake of convenience, it's great to have a little stair machine all to ourselves.

The Nordic Track Machine

The Nordic Track machine is another wonderful home exercise invention. It too can be purchased at a reasonable price. Its advantage over the stationary bicycle or even the stair machine is that it challenges the upper body as well as the lower body. You really get total-body stimulation when you exercise with the Nordic Track machine. Your chest, shoulders, back, arms, legs, and buttocks are working all the time.

You can purchase the Nordic Track machine in many sporting goods or department stores.

Walking Fast

Walking is almost as good as running, if you do it fast and for double the length of time. I've experimented with running twenty minutes five times a week, then substituted walking forty minutes at a brisk pace, five times a week. After doing each one for six months, I found that the walking seemed to help me burn more fat than did the running. I believe this has to do with the fact that I doubled my walking time. You probably do not need to double your time when walking to get the same fat-burning effect as running for twenty minutes. Perhaps you only have to increase your time by one-third if you want to walk instead of run. However, since there is no proof of this yet, if you choose to walk instead of run, jump, or bike, double your time just to be on the safe side.

I usually do my walking during the natural course of a work day. For example, in New York City, rather than take the bus or subway, I wear my running shoes with my business suit and carry my high heels in my briefcase. I will walk anywhere from twenty to forty minutes. By the time I arrive at my destination, I am refreshed and ready to deal with the issues at hand.

If you are going to walk to a business destination, you should dress a little lighter than you would if you were going to drive or take public transportation. That way you won't arrive with your makeup running or your clothing sticking to your body.

OTHER AEROBIC ACTIVITIES

There are a variety of aerobic activities not mentioned above that can be used to burn extra fat. Aerobic dancing, swimming, cross-country skiing, tennis, raquetball, and squash, to name a few. Whatever activity you choose, remember to work at it in a vigorous manner. The more energy you put into it, the more fat you will burn. And remember, don't feel that if you can't do it for a full twenty minutes that it's a waste of time. Everything counts. Even if you only have ten to fifteen minutes to spare, do it anyway. It all adds up.

Here is a chart designating the approximate amount of calories you will burn if you engage in the indicated activity for twenty minutes.

AEROBIC EXERCISE CHART

Aerobic Activity	Calories Burned per 20 Minutes
Stair machine	260
Running	220
Cross-country skiing	220
Swimming	210
Rope jumping	200
Aerobic dance	200
Race walking	160
Squash	160
Bicycle riding	140
Walking	110

The above calculations are based upon the assumption that you maintain a moderate pace. If you tense your muscles as you're exercising, if you go a little faster, and/or if you work a little harder, of course you will burn more calories than the chart indicates. On the other hand, if you behave as if you're about to fall asleep as you go, you will burn fewer calories than the chart indicates.

HOW TO BURN FAT DURING THE TYPICAL WORKDAY

Perhaps like most people you are so busy that you don't always have time to fit in an aerobic activity. For you, it is especially important to learn to utilize natural opportunities to get your body moving.

If you think about it, there are several clear openings during the course of a typical workday that can be used to burn some additional fat. The idea is to put your body in motion—to break the habit of sitting in one spot and vegetating. Here are some ideas.

Stand up! If you have a sedentary desk job, make it your business to stand at least half the time you would otherwise be sitting. For example, when you are talking on the telephone, you could stand up and pace a little. Get yourself an extension cord if you don't already have one. Instead of calling into the next office or across the room, get up and go speak to the person there. Move from point A to point B. Every time you move, you energize yourself. You force your metabolism to go into action, to wake up, to help you burn more fat.

Take short walks during the day. Park your car ten minutes away from work. If you take public transportation to work, you can make it your business to get off the bus or train a ten- to twenty-minute walk away from work. If you can't or won't do that, take a short walk before or after lunch.

Walk ten minutes after every meal. After you eat, instead of sitting down to read the paper or watch television, go outside and take a brisk walk for ten minutes. It won't kill you, and you'll feel energized when you return. The walk will have speeded up your metabolism so that some of the calories you have just eaten will quickly be gone. The walk will also help your digestion process. In addition, instead of feeling lethargic and sleepy, as one often feels just after eating, you will feel awake and alive. You might even get some chores done that you otherwise would have neglected.

Use the stairs rather than the elevator. It will save you time (the elevator is usually crowded) and will provide you with an excellent aerobic spurt. The first time you try this (unless you have been climbing stairs or using the stair

188

machine), you may feel a bit out of breath. After you get used to it, it will be a breeze. If you have on tight clothing, you will be more out of breath than usual, but don't worry; you'll burn those calories just the same. So do it. If you are wearing high heels, you can still climb the stairs; just go a little slower. No excuses. Get that exercise in. A little here, a little there, a little less fat.

Take an exercise coffee break. Instead of sitting around and talking on your coffee break, do the 12-Minute Total-Body Workout (see the bibliography). You'll go back to your desk feeling energized and in a much better mood. You can always have your coffee at your desk.

THINGS TO WATCH FOR AT HOME

■ **Don't languish for hours in front of the television.** Most of us work very hard during the day, and we deserve to relax when we come home. There's nothing wrong with lounging on the couch and watching some favorite television programs after a long day at the office. But don't lie on the couch for more than an hour. Force yourself to get up and move around the house. Do an annoying chore during a commercial or between programs—the dishes, vacuum cleaning, or dusting. You'll be surprised to find that where before you thought you had no energy and were about to doze off, now, after doing the chore, you feel awake and alert.

What happened? You sparked your sleepy metabolism and it's now in gear. You will now be burning additional calories for the next hour or two just because you got up and moved around.

■ **Don't put something in your mouth every five minutes.** When at home, it's tempting to take regular walks to the refrigerator out of sheer boredom. You can check yourself by making a simple rule. After you've eaten dinner, you will *not* go to the refrigerator for at least two hours. Then, you will go only once in an hour. And even when you do go to the refrigerator, you will keep within the bounds of the eating plan you are following, either for weight (fat) loss or maintenance.

- **Don't eat while standing at the refrigerator.** Most of us do that. We stand at the refrigerator when no one is around and consume whatever is there, without the use of knife, fork, or spoon. We don't care, because no one is around to see us. All well and good, but there's a problem: The food we gulp down is digested and processed and added up in calories for use or storage as fat, even though no one was there to observe the act.

In short, it's easy to eat too much while enjoying these furtive binges. For this reason, you have to make it a rule that you won't put anything in your mouth unless you are sitting down and have the food on a plate.

- **Don't eat while talking on the telephone.** Besides the fact that it's rude (they really can hear you chewing, even if you hold the mouthpiece up from time to time), it's very difficult to monitor the amount of food you're eating. The only exception I will make to this rule is in a case where you are really in a rush, and you would otherwise have to skip a meal.

- **Be aware that you are eating if you want to enjoy a meal while watching television or reading the paper.** You've probably been warned not to eat while watching television or reading the paper, but, quite frankly, that's ridiculous. You deserve to enjoy yourself and relax in any fashion that pleases you while you eat. The only danger in watching television or reading the paper while eating is that you can eat too much if you are unaware of what you are doing. The way to avoid this is to acknowledge mentally that the portion you serve yourself is indeed your meal, and that you will not be going back for seconds, thirds, and fourths. If you do this, you can enjoy your food fully while at the same time unwinding and amusing yourself. It's quite an enjoyable thing to do, and I do it quite often.

Of course, it is always better to share a dinner with a wonderful friend and to take two hours to complete the meal as you fully savor the food. But this isn't always possible.

PERFECTING TROUBLESOME BODY PARTS

If you have a specific body part that really bothers you, here's what you can do. (You may use any or all of these suggestions.)

1. If you are not already using the Insanity plan, use it for your troublesome body part(s).

2. Instead of doing three sets for each of the exercises for the troublesome body part(s), do four. Here's how your workout will look:

   Set 1: fifteen repetitions with three-pound dumbbells
   Set 2: twelve repetitions with five-pound dumbbells
   Set 3: ten repetitions with eight-pound dumbbells
   Set 4: eight repetitions with ten-pound dumbbells

   (You may lower or raise the weights according to your present level of strength.)

3. Instead of working out the minimum of three days per week for the troublesome body part(s), work out the maximum of five days per week for the body part(s). In other words, if you are now working out three days a week with the regular program, add in two more days, but only for your troublesome body part(s). Be sure to observe the "split routine" system. The exception to this rule is buttocks and abdominals, which can be exercised two days in a row.

4. Do not take advantage of the ten- to fifteen-second rest periods when exercising your troublesome body part(s). Instead, complete the entire exercise group for that body part before resting. (You will have to break in gently in order to do this. It may take you a few months.)

5. For buttocks and abdominals, increase your repetitions to fifty per set.

6. For buttocks and abdominals, use the additional light weight discussed in the "alternatives" section.

7. For thighs, increase all of your repetitions to fifteen per set, but continue to use the modified pyramid system.

8. Add in a sixth and even seventh exercise for your troublesome body part. (See the alternatives indicated with exercises for the various body parts.)

9. Apply continuous tension by squeezing the working muscle as hard as possible throughout the exercise, both on the up and down movement, while still maintaining your pace.

If you put in the extra time and energy, you will see results that much more quickly. But make sure you are physically capable of the challenge. As mentioned in the opening pages of this book, it is important to check with your doctor before undertaking any new exercise program.

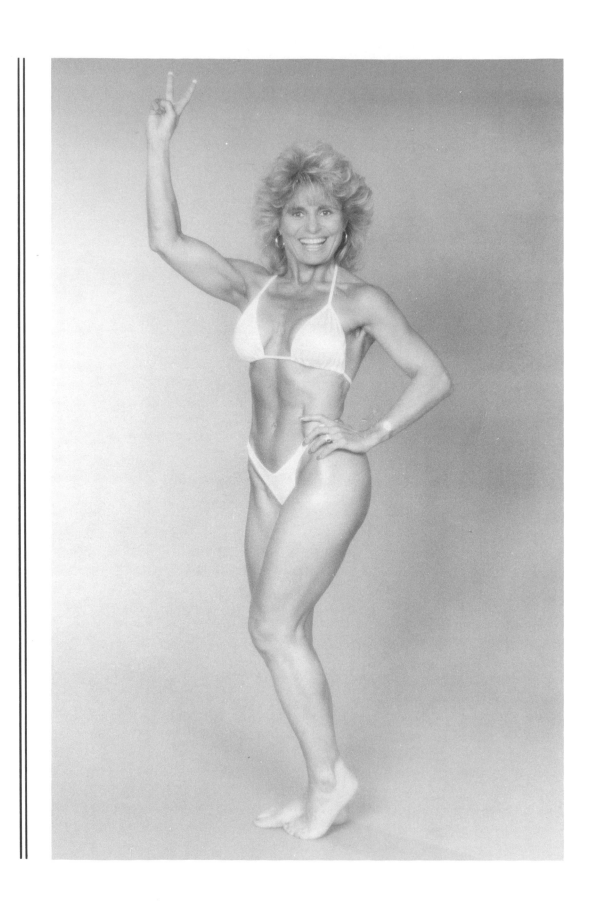

10 | KEEPING IT OFF AND SHOWING IT OFF

Getting it off is one thing. Keeping it off is another. In this chapter, you will learn how to maintain your fat-loss and keep your shapely body. You'll be pleased to find out that you don't have to continue to do the Fat-Burning Workout all year round. You can choose any one of the maintenance plans.

What good is it to get the fat off and reshape your body if you never get the chance to show it off? What's more, isn't it a shame to be in great shape and then wear a bathing suit that emphasizes your hips and makes you look ten pounds fatter than you really are?

By the time you finish reading the following paragraphs you will be well prepared to enjoy your beautiful body every day of your life.

NOW THAT YOU GOT IT OFF, HOW CAN YOU KEEP IT OFF?

You might think that once you get in shape, you can rest on your laurels and relax. You have nothing to worry about. The fat will never come back. *Wrong*. Of course you will have to do something to maintain your new body. But there is good news. You won't have to work as hard as you did to get that new body.

Although you may have gotten into shape in four to six weeks by using the

Fat-Burning Workout, I suggest that you continue to do the workout for at least six months. After that you may continue with the workout or switch to one of the alternate programs discussed in the following paragraphs.

■ **Do the Fat-Burning Workout all year round or until you can't take it any more.**

You can continue to do the Fat-Burning Workout forever. Perhaps you enjoy it, even though it is quite intense. You may decide to switch to the plan that requires the least work (the regular Fat-Burning Workout) if you were doing the Intensity or Insanity workout. You may also decide to do the workout three or four days a week if you were putting in the maximum of five days. It's up to you.

However, after a while, chances are you may feel the need for a change of pace. Your body may tell you to try something different. When this happens, it's a good idea to pay attention to the feeling. Otherwise you may be tempted to stop working out altogether.

Once you realize that it's time for a change, select from one or a combination of the following workout plans.

■ **Switch to a regular exercise plan for nine months of the year. Do the Fat-Burning Workout only three months of the year.**

If you want to do this, you have two choices. You can use this book with the modifications indicated below, or you can get a copy of my regular weight-training book, *Now or Never*. If you use this book, here is what you will have to do in order to convert the program into a regular body-shaping program.

First, you will no longer do giant, super-giant, or monster sets. Instead, you will perform your exercises in the manner of a regular body-building routine. In order to do this, you will have to complete each exercise for a given body part before proceeding to the next exercise for that body part, and you will have to rest thirty to forty-five seconds between sets. In addition, you will have to use slightly higher weights—as heavy a weight as you can handle and still get the required number of repetitions.

Using the biceps routine as an example, you will do your first set of twelve repetitions of your first biceps exercise, the standing alternate dumbbell curl, with ten-pound dumbbells. You will rest for thirty to forty-five seconds, and then do your second set of ten repetitions of that exercise with fifteen-pound dumbbells. You will again rest for thirty to forty-five seconds before proceeding to your final set of eight repetitions with twenty-pound dumbbells. Then, and only then, will you proceed to your next biceps exercise, the standing angled simultaneous dumbbell curl, after again having rested thirty to forty-five seconds. For further review of the difference between regular weight training and super-giant and monster setting, see chapter 5.

When you turn the Fat-Burning Workout into a regular body-shaping routine, you will still have to decide whether you want to do three, four, or five exercises per body part. If in doubt, take the middle road and do four exercises per body part. Also realize that your workout will now take you about twice as long as before, since you will be resting for greater periods of time.

Since working with weights in a regular body-building routine does not yield an aerobic effect, it will be necessary to do at least three twenty-minute aerobic sessions or three forty-minute walking sessions per week in addition to the program. It is not optional in this case.

- **Do the 12-Minute Total-Body Workout for nine months of the year. Use the Fat-Burning Workout when needed.**

The 12-Minute Total-Body Workout is great if you want a real change of pace and a seeming vacation from working out. With this routine, you only have to work out twelve minutes a day, but you do have to work out every day—there are no days off—and the workout is very intense. You exercise three body parts a day, and you do three sets of ten repetitions for each exercise. But you must apply continual pressure to the working muscle. The workout causes your muscles to become dense and defined, but you cannot add any size to your muscles this way.

For those of you who do not wish to purchase *The 12-Minute Total-Body Workout*, here is a way to convert the Fat-Burning Workout to a twelve-minute plan. Exercise three body parts every day. Do only two exercises per body part. (You may pick from any of the exercises presented in this book.) Do three sets of ten repetitions for each exercise, using three-pound dumbbells, and squeeze your working muscle as hard as possible as you work, both on the stretch and flex part of the exercise. (The applying of pressure on the stretch part of the exercise is called "dynamic tension." The squeezing of the muscle on the flex part of the exercise is called "isometric pressure.")

After six days, you will have exercised all nine body parts twice, and you will have one day left. On this day, you will exercise your buttocks and abdominals a third time, since these are the body parts that tend to attract fat.

In addition to this workout, you will have to do at least three twenty-minute aerobic sessions, or three forty-minute walking sessions. Since this workout does not yield an aerobic effect, the additional aerobics are not optional.

- **Switch from the Fat-Burning Workout to the Now or Never Workout or the 12-Minute Workout as your body demands.**

The best plan is to switch on and off between all three methods during the course of the year. You may tune in to the needs of your own body and switch as you see fit. Here are some possibilities.

1. Change plans every four months. Do the Fat-Burning Workout for four months, then regular weight training as shown in *Now or Never* for four months, then a daily twelve-minute plan as demonstrated in the *12-Minute Total-Body Workout* for three months.

2. Change plans in accordance with the seasons. Do the Fat-Burning Workout in the spring and summer, to remain lean and mean for the summer months, then switch to a twelve-minute plan for the fall and winter months.

3. Change plans when you want to build bigger muscles. Do the Fat-Burning Workout until you get rid of all of your excess body fat. Then switch to regular weight training in order to build slightly larger muscles.

4. Change plans in order to build up one specific body part. You may switch to a regular weight training program as described above, just for that body part, and continue to do the Fat-Burning Workout for all of your other body parts, or you can get a copy of *Perfect Parts* and follow the routine described in that book for the body part you want to develop.

5. Switch from one plan to the other (Fat-Burning Workout, regular bodybuilding, a twelve-minute routine, or special body-shaping) at will, whenever your body tells you to or whenever you become bored with the routine you are doing.

ADDITIONAL AEROBICS

Use additional aerobic activities whenever you see too much fat on your body. In order to maintain your fat-free shapely body, you'll have to keep your eyes open when you look in the mirror. If you notice that you are seeing a little more fat than usual, it's a good idea immediately to incorporate some aerobic activities into your weekly routine, before the fat becomes a problem. Start out by doing three twenty-minute sessions a week and build up to five thirty-minute sessions if necessary. Better yet, start walking every day for thirty to forty minutes. You'll see a difference in a matter of weeks. The whole idea of maintaining fat loss is to catch the regaining cycle before it gets out of hand. Why wait until you are ten pounds too fat and have to go on a really strict regimen?

SOME WEIGHT FLUCTUATION IS NORMAL

If you find you go up and down the scale seasonally, don't panic.

It's important to realize that the human body does not usually stay at the same weight all year round. Most people gain a few pounds (three to seven) in the winter, not because they are naughty and throw all caution to the wind, but because in the winter the body responds to the colder weather by slowing down the metabolism in order to build up an insulating layer of fat for protection against the cold.

The body is not vain. It's a survival system. It could care less that you do not like the way it looks with the additional adipose (fat) tissue, nor does it appreciate the fact that you do not respect its efforts to help you to survive a cold winter, and that you are trying to work against it by forcing it to eat less and work harder. In fact, your body may put up quite a fight if you try to lose that last bit of lingering fat during the cold weather.

Don't misunderstand or use this as an excuse to wait until the warmer months to start your fitness regimen. Although it is usually more difficult to lose weight in the colder months than during the warmer season, it is not impossible. It can be done and, as a matter of fact, it is done all the time. People lose weight and get in shape all year round.

Every winter, I regularly gain about seven pounds. I've learned not to panic. I don't look "fat" with the added seven pounds because I'm in shape. I just look bigger. Unless I'm preparing for a photo shoot or a television show, I've learned to let my body weight run its natural winter course, and I don't trouble myself with diets or intense workout plans. I have found through experience that this isn't necessary, because when springtime rolls around, my metabolism speeds up, I become more energetic, and with just a little extra push on my part, I shed the added weight.

I can imagine what you're thinking now. "Seven pounds—that's a lot of weight." Yes it is. Before I knew that losing and gaining weight is really based upon laws of nature, I used to panic the moment I gained a few pounds. I thought I would never get them off. I worried that no matter what I did I would continue to gain weight until I was as fat as a house. So I would immediately launch a drastic weight-loss or starvation diet program, which, by the way, usually failed. I'm much calmer about losing and gaining weight now that I realize there is no mystery about the whole procedure. The body loses and gains weight according to a clearly defined scientific process.

If you cut down on your calories, increase your activity, and work to speed up your metabolism by exercising and adding muscle to your body, in time you will lose the weight. It's that simple. There's no more reason to doubt that it will work than there is to question the law of gravity. When I drop a pencil, I have no fear that it will fly upward. I know that it will fall to the ground. The only difference is, it's easier to believe in the law of gravity than it is to believe in the science of losing and gaining weight, because the law of gravity is demonstrated instantly. The loss and gain of weight is demonstrated over time. For this reason, we are momentarily required to have faith, as it were, and to believe in something that we cannot immediately see, although intellectually we know it to be true.

GIVE YOURSELF A MOTIVE TO KEEP IT OFF

Sometimes it's hard to keep the fat off your body and to stay in shape if you have no special motivation. True, you got in shape for yourself—so that you could feel happy, proud, healthy, and no longer ashamed of your body—but now that you have reached your goal, you may feel a bit let down.

Why is this so? Perhaps unconsciously you were thinking that after you lost the weight, your life would miraculously change for the better. And yet there you are—in your same house, the same old Lisa, Jane, or Joan. Where is all the adventure that you expected would suddenly come to you?

The simple fact is, you have to make your own adventure, create your own excitement. Rather than slip back into old habits of inactivity and overindulgence, you must make a conscious effort to find something to get excited about.

Whether you are married or unattached, here are some suggestions that will help to keep you motivated to stay in shape. I regularly use a combination of all of them.

■ **Take frequent, short vacations where you will be seen in a bathing suit.** Perhaps this is the best way to keep yourself motivated—a frequent reward of sun and fun. Just when you were thinking of hibernating like a bear and piling on a thick layer of fat, you realize that in three weeks you will be going to Mexico in the dead of your winter. So instead of falling into the malaise of aimless eating, you step up your workout program and watch your diet so that you can "strut your stuff" on the beach.

■ **Work toward a special occasion.** Think of special occasions where you will be meeting people whom you would like to impress with your wonderful body. It could be a family holiday gathering, a class reunion, or a date with an old friend. If no such gathering or meeting is about to take place, make one happen by setting it up yourself. What is wrong with calling an old friend, male or female, and asking that person out to lunch in three weeks? Then motivate yourself not only to maintain your present fit body for that occasion, but to improve yourself even further for the event. When that meeting is over, set up another date with family or friends. You have the power to make your life work. It's up to you to use it.

- **Engage a photographer.** That's right—hire a special photographer to take a series of photographs of your beautiful new body. You can set up a photo shoot for three months from a given date, then make it your business to refine your body into its most perfect form for that date.

Not only will you have given yourself a motive to remain in shape for that date, but once you have the photographs, you can use them to inspire yourself to remain in shape. This photo shoot could take place every two years, and then you could see that, indeed, you are not getting older, you are getting better. If you follow the fitness plan outlined in this book, you will look better every year. I'm forty-seven years old now, and I look better than I did at twenty-seven and thirty-seven. I feel better, too.

- **Enter a fitness, beauty, or bodybuilders' contest.** Now, don't throw this book across the room. I'm not suggesting that you aim at winning the contest. I'm merely asking you to enter a contest just for the fun of it. It doesn't cost anything, and if you pick an amateur contest, the rules for entry are generally minimal. Anyone can sign up. Wouldn't it be fun to sashay across the stage behaving like a beauty queen? Who cares if you come in last place? (I did come in last once when I entered a contest and I lived. In fact, it was funny.)

You can find contests to enter by inquiring at local gyms and health spas. Some contests are geared more toward bodybuilding than fitness. But even if you entered a bodybuilding contest, it wouldn't matter. Your goal is to be beautiful. So what if you lose because your muscles are not as big as those of the other ladies? You will have won a contest with yourself—a dare to take a chance and do something different

- **Get involved in a romantic relationship.** We all know that one of the best motivations for not allowing that lower stomach to return to the status of "little pot," or for refusing to let the cellulite return to the thighs and the saddle bags to the hips, is often the love interest in our lives. We remember all too well the days when we lived in fear of being seen in the nude, when we scrambled to turn off the lights whenever an intimate situation arose, and when we constantly apologized for our bodies. We recall living in dread of a comment being made about our unsightly body parts. So every time we think about slacking off on our fitness program and letting our body return to its former state, a love interest prompts us to dismiss the thought quickly and continue to work hard at keeping in shape.

Now that I think of it, I have a recommendation for all single women. If you haven't been involved in a relationship in over a year, it's time to flirt a little.

Of course, if you enjoy your solitude and are not in the mood to deal with anyone at this point, there are other alternatives.

OTHER WAYS TO HELP YOURSELF STAY IN SHAPE

Learn to treat yourself with love and care. Pamper and respect yourself. Here are some ideas.

- **Go to a luxurious health spa.** Just when you're feeling down and out, instead of allowing yourself to sink deeper into despair, pick up the telephone and make a reservation at a health spa. (See the bibliography for a book that will help you to make your selection—*The Ultimate Spa Book.*) Allow yourself to be pampered and taken care of for a few days or even a week. You'll come back feeling like a new person, and your motivation to stay trim and healthy will have multiplied. Don't feel guilty about spending the money. You deserve the luxury. You only go around once. If you don't take care of yourself, who will?

- **Buy designer clothing.** Clothing may not make the man or woman, but it certainly does have the power to make the man or woman feel elegant. Think of a designer whose name you've always known and whose clothing line you've always admired. Then take a special trip to a shop where that designer's clothing is featured. Spend the day trying on various outfits. If you see something you love, buy it on the spot. Be frivolous. But don't stop there. Your next step will be to . . .

- **Consult a fashion expert.** Go to a high-fashion department store such as Saks Fifth Avenue. Ask for the fashion coordinator or shopping service. If you choose Saks Fifth Avenue, they will send you to the Fifth Avenue Club, where they have special fashion consultants. These people will sit you down and offer you a Perrier while they have their people run all over the store in search of items that will look great on you. All you have to do is tell them what kind of outfit you are interested in. They will return with full outfits in a choice of sizes, complete with accessories—from shoes, hose, and handbag to jewelry—and yes, even underwear if you choose.

These people are marvelous. And what's more, they will not allow you to leave the store with anything that does not suit you exactly. In addition, they can be counted on to outfit you for any and every possible occasion, with the guarantee that you will be elegantly and appropriately dressed. There is no charge for this service. You'll walk out of the store feeling like a million dollars.

- **Consult a hair and makeup specialist.** When is the last time you changed your hairstyle? How do you know that the look you have been wearing is the most flattering to your face? Have you been doing your makeup a certain way for years? It's time for a change. Let the experts have a go at you. Look in your local telephone directory under beauty consultants, or call a major photographer. If you call a photographer, tell him that your goal is a hairstyle change and a makeup consultation. Ask if he can recommend any of his hair and makeup people. Chances are, he'll take your number and speak to one of his best assistants. That person will call you, and the two of you can work out your own deal.

These people are experts. They often work with models, television and movie stars, and professionals whose livelihood depends upon their image. With their help, you can bring out your natural beauty and, by following their advice, maintain it. It takes courage to even think of change. I challenge you to do it.

LEARN HOW TO WEAR A BATHING SUIT AND HOW TO POSE IN ONE

Unfortunately, many people take one step forward and two steps back when it comes to looking their best. They spend months getting into shape, and then, when it comes time to showcase the results of their hard work, they choose the worst possible styles in clothing to show it off.

Most likely, the reason for this is simple ignorance. Most of us did not take a course in fashion design and body contour, so we do the best we can when it comes to style. I'm not going to try to give a crash course here, but I will help you with the most revealing aspect of dress, the bathing suit, because once you get in shape, that's what you'll be wearing more often than ever before, and why shouldn't you look your best when you do?

Picking the Bathing Suit

The first decision is whether to wear a one- or two-piece bathing suit. If your stomach is still a little paunchy, it may be a good idea to opt for the one piece. If you do, make sure the suit has high-cut legs rather than legs cut straight across. Also, select a style that is low-cut on the sides (under the arms) rather than high-cut. This kind of suit will help you look your slimmest.

If you choose a two-piece bathing suit, don't wear it straight across your hips. That will not only make your hips appear wider, but will also create a "lump" where the strap cuts into your hip. (See my "wrong" picture, p. 203.) Instead, pull the sides up as high as you can so that a "V" look is effected, and the natural curve of your hip-thigh is not interrupted. (See my "right" picture, p. 203.) Also, make sure you don't choose a suit that is cut straight across the leg or is cut too high on the waist. This will make you look boxy and bulky.

202

Now let's talk about the top. If you choose to wear a strapless top, unless it is boned, or you have large, high breasts, you will either have to pay constant dilligence to your pulling your shoulders back (the way I am in my "right" photograph on p. 203) or look the way I do in my "wrong" photograph. It's better to choose a low-cut style with straps, one that clearly separates your breasts. (See opening chapter shot, chapter 10.)

Posture and Posing

Have the "wrong" and "right" photographs in front of you as you read this (p. 203). If you're out to put your best look on in a bathing suit, instead of standing full-front with your stomach out and your shoulders stooped and your feet pointed outward, twist your body to the side, pull your stomach in, draw your shoulders back and keep your feet close together, bending one leg. This stance will give you your most flattering body line. Look at the difference my stance makes in the photographs. You would think I were ten pounds heavier in the "wrong" photograph, yet both pictures were taken in the same bathing suit, ten minutes apart, on the same day.

Don't take my word for it. Have some fun yourself by taking "wrong" and "right" photographs of your own, and see the difference these few pointers can make.

Bathing Footwear

Do yourself a favor and throw away those flat-footed thongs. They're extremely unflattering. Also discard the ultra high heels. You will look too much like a Las Vegas showgirl. Instead, choose a simple slip-on sandal with a two- or three-inch stacked heel.

MUSCLES CAN HIDE THE FAT

Notice by looking at my pictures that I have developed lines of definition on two places on my body. These lines serve to draw attention away from broad areas, making my body appear slimmer and shapelier than it really is.

Look at the definition in my upper back muscles. This definition helps to draw attention away from my large buttocks. It helps to balance out my total

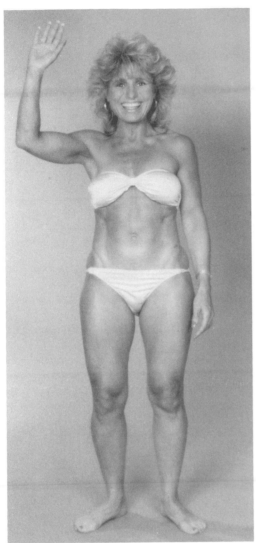

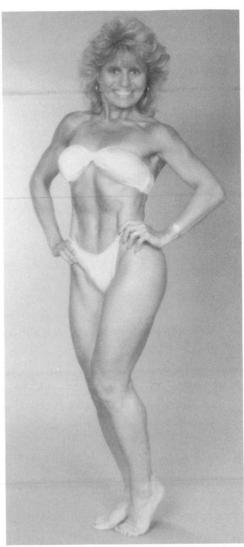

Wrong way to wear a bathing suit
and pose

Right way to wear a bathing suit
and pose

body look by bringing the eye up and away from my derriere. I achieved the muscles and the definition by doing pee-wee laterals and seated and lying dumbbell back laterals.

Look at my waist. Even though it measures twenty-seven inches (not very small, by any account) it appears much smaller. What makes my waist look smaller are the lines of definition running along my side abdominals. These are the external oblique muscles, and the lines of definition were achieved by doing the serratus pull. See front anatomy photo on p. 45.

The creation of muscles and definition in one area of the body to balance out or offset the muscles or body shape in another area, or to create an illusion, has been used by bodybuilders for many years. Now you can take advantage of these methods to perfect your own body.

You will naturally attain these muscles in a matter of weeks or months as you faithfully follow the Fat-Burning Workout. However, if you want to speed up your progress or emphasize these muscles to a greater extent, you may do extra work on specific body parts by choosing among the methods discussed in chapter 9.

REMINDERS

If you want to stay in shape, and look in shape, here are some reminders.

1. It's not over once you get in shape. You can't just let your body lie stagnant. Choose a maintenance plan and stick to it. You may change plans as often as you please.

2. It's okay to gain weight (up to seven pounds) in the wintertime. Don't panic. Your body will be ready to shed the extra weight when the warmer weather comes around.

3. In order to stay in shape, you'll need motivation. There are many exciting ways to motivate yourself.

4. Be good to yourself. Treat yourself to designer clothing. Consult experts in hair, makeup and fashion. Go to a health spa. Love yourself.

5. Choose a bathing suit that will flatter your figure.

6. Be alert to your posture when wearing a bikini. Pull your stomach in and your shoulders back. Stand high on your toes and twist your body to the side.

7. If you have big hips and a big waist, take advantage of bodybuilding tricks to draw attention away from these areas. You can place lines of definition in certain strategic places.

I'm interested in hearing from you. If you want to write to me to discuss your progress or to ask a question, feel free to do so. If you wish an answer, please *include a stamped, self-addressed envelope.*

If you wish to order workout equipment, or a personally autographed black-and-white or color glossy photograph of me, send a check or money order for the designated price to the address listed below (U.S. currency only). You will be billed for the UPS shipping of the dumbbells and exercise bench (COD). There will be no additional shipping charge for the photographs, which will be sent by the U.S. postal service. We are unable to ship to Canada.

CAST-IRON DUMBBELLS
(as seen in exercise photographs)

Set of 3- pound dumbbells $12.98
Set of 5- pound dumbbells $17.98
Set of 8- pound dumbbells $24.98
Set of 10- pound dumbbells $29.98
Set of 12- pound dumbbells $34.98
Set of 15- pound dumbbells $39.98

(You pay UPS shipping charges, COD.)

FLAT-INCLINE STEEL UPHOLSTERED EXERCISE BENCH $139.98
(You pay UPS shipping charges, COD)

8 X 10 BLACK AND WHITE GLOSSY
PERSONALLY AUTOGRAPHED PHOTOGRAPH $10.00
COLOR PHOTOGRAPH $12.00

(I pay shipping charges.) Photographs mailed by U.S. mail.

Address all correspondence to:

Joyce L. Vedral
P.O. Box A433
Wantagh, NY 11793–0433

Good luck. I'm with you all the way.

BIBLIOGRAPHY

NUTRITION BOOKS
FOR ADDITIONAL INFORMATION

Hausman, Patricia, M.S. *The Calcium Bible.* New York: Rawson Associates, 1985.

Eades, Michael R., M.D. *Thin So Fast.* New York: Warner Books, 1989.

Giller, Robert M., M.D., and Kathy Matthews. *Maximum Metabolism.* New York: G. P. Putnam's Sons, 1989.

Katahn, Martin, Ph.D. *The T-Factor Diet.* New York: W. W. Norton & Company, 1989.

Kirshbaum, John (ed.). *The Nutrition Almanac.* New York: McGraw-Hill, 1989.

Reynolds, Bill, and Joyce L. Vedral, Ph.D. *Supercut: Nutrition for the Ultimate Physique.* Chicago: Contemporary Books, 1985.

Spear, Ruth. *Low Fat and Loving It: How to Lower Your Fat Intake and Still Eat the Foods You Love—200 Delicious Recipes.* New York: Warner Books, 1991.

EXERCISE BOOKS
FOR ADDITIONAL TRAINING

Francis, Bev. *Power Bodybuilding*. New York: Sterling Books, 1989.

Kneuer, Cameo, and Joyce L. Vedral, Ph.D. *Cameo Fitness*. New York: Warner Books, 1990.

McLish, Rachel, and Joyce L. Vedral, Ph.D. *Perfect Parts*. New York: Warner Books, 1987.

Portugues, Gladys, and Joyce L. Vedral, Ph.D. *Hard Bodies*. New York: Dell Publishing, 1986.

Portugues, Gladys, and Joyce L. Vedral, Ph.D. *Hard Bodies Express Workout*. New York: Dell Publishing, 1988.

Vedral, Joyce, Ph.D. *Now or Never*. New York: Warner Books, 1986.

Vedral, Joyce, Ph.D. *The 12-Minute Total-Body Workout*. New York: Warner Books, 1989.

MAGAZINES FOR EXERCISE
AND NUTRITIONAL INFORMATION

American Health, 80 Fifth Avenue, New York, NY 10011

Longevity, 1965 Broadway, New York, NY 10023–5965

Female Bodybuilding, 351 East 84th Street, New York, NY 10028

Muscle and Fitness, 21100 Erwin Street, Woodland Hills, CA 91367

Shape, 21100 Erwin Street, Woodland Hills, CA 91367

Your Health, 540 N.W. Broken Sound Blvd., Boca Raton, FL 33431

208

NEWSLETTERS
FOR NUTRITIONAL INFORMATION

Mayo Clinic Nutrition Letter, 200 First Street, S.W., Rochester, MN 55905

Tufts University Diet and Nutrition Letter, P.O. Box 57857, Boulder, CO 80322–7857

University of California, Berkeley, Wellness Letter, Health Letter Associates, P.O. Box 420148, Palm Coast, FL 32142

OTHER BOOKS FOR HELPFUL INFORMATION

Borysenko, Joan, Ph.D. *Minding the Body, Mending the Mind*. Reading, Massachusetts: Addison-Wesley Publishing, 1987.

Borysenko, Joan, Ph.D. *Guilt Is the Teacher, Love Is the Lesson*. New York: Warner Books, 1990.

Ornstein, Robert, Ph.D., and David Sobel, M.D. *The Healing Brain*. New York: Simon and Schuster, 1987.

INDEX